Authors' Acknowledgments

From Joanne: I want to thank my husband, Tim, for his never-ending support and encouragement for me to do whatever I need to be happy . . . even if that means everything else becomes "just too much" before a deadline.

To Ava, I thank you for sharing your beautiful smile in Mommy's book.

Thank you to my subs, Ginger, Jillian, and Mariah, for giving Ava loving and nurturing care when I needed to write and she needed to squeak and play.

To my coauthor, Ilene — without your experience and knowledge, we couldn't have written this book. It has been my pleasure to get to know you better — thank you.

To Anna Damaskos, for giving my name to Grace Freedson, thank you; and to Grace, my literary agent, thank you for your support in getting this project.

To Joan Friedman, our project editor, I want to say that I couldn't ask for a better editor — thank you.

Thank you to Kathryn Born and Margie Pillar for the beautiful illustrations and photographs.

To my family, friends, and Core Community: Each of you, in your unique way, helps me reach for the stars.

From Ilene: Terence, I want to thank you for putting up with me for the past eight-plus years, for being my massage subject when I was still a student and didn't know what I was doing, and for your support when I thought I couldn't do it.

To my clients, I want to say that I appreciate you giving me the honor of working with you. Because of your receptivity and our shared wisdom, we have the opportunity to learn how we can heal ourselves through the power of touch: with compassion, care, presence and tenderness.

Thank you, Joanne, for making this possible with all your hard work and determination. To Ava, thank you for being so good-natured all the time.

Thank you to all the babies, my parents, and my friends.

D1304352

Publisher's Acknowledgments

We're proud of this book; please send us your comments through our Dummies online registration form located at www.dummies.com/register/.

Some of the people who helped bring this book to market include the following:

Acquisitions, Editorial, and Media Development

Project Editor: Joan Friedman

Acquisitions Editor: Tracy Boggier

Technical Editors: Laura Tucker Guzzi, Julie Bittner Miller

Editorial Manager: Michelle Hacker

Editorial Supervisor: Carmen Krikorian

Editorial Assistants: Courtney Allen, Nadine Bell

Cover Photos: © Tracy Boggier/2004

Cartoons: Rich Tennant, www.the5thwave.com

Composition

Project Coordinator: Adrienne Martinez

Layout and Graphics: Andrea Dahl, Lauren Goddard, Barry Offringa, Jacque Roth, Heather Ryan

Special Art: Interior photographs by Marjorie S. Pillar; Illustrations by Kathryn Born, MA

Proofreaders: Leeann Harney, Jessica Kramer, Carl William Pierce, TECHBOOKS Production Services

Indexer: TECHBOOKS Production Services

Publishing and Editorial for Consumer Dummies

Diane Graves Steele, Vice President and Publisher, Consumer Dummies

Joyce Pepple, Acquisitions Director, Consumer Dummies

Kristin A. Cocks, Product Development Director, Consumer Dummies

Michael Spring, Vice President and Publisher, Travel

Brice Gosnell, Associate Publisher, Travel

Kelly Regan, Editorial Director, Travel

Publishing for Technology Dummies

Andy Cummings, Vice President and Publisher, Dummies Technology/General User

Composition Services

Gerry Fahey, Vice President of Production Services

Debbie Stailey, Director of Composition Services

Baby Massage

FOR

DUMMIES®

Baby Massage

FOR

DUMMIES

By Joanne Bagshaw, M.A., and Ilene Fox

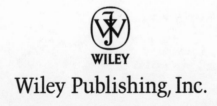

WILEY

Wiley Publishing, Inc.

Baby Massage For Dummies®

Published by
Wiley Publishing, Inc.
111 River St.
Hoboken, NJ 07030-5774
www.wiley.com

For general information on our other products and services, please contact our Customer Care Department within the U.S. at 800-762-2974, outside the U.S. at 317-572-3993, or fax 317-572-4002.

For technical support, please visit www.wiley.com/techsupport.

Wiley also publishes its books in a variety of electronic formats. Some content that appears in print may not be available in electronic books.

Library of Congress Control Number: 2004117446

ISBN: 0-7645-7841-3

Manufactured in the United States of America

10 9 8 7 6 5 4 3 2 1

1B/QS/QS/QV/IN

WILEY

About the Authors

Joanne Bagshaw is a psychotherapist, writer, and promoter of attachment parenting. She has a master's degree in Forensic Psychology from John Jay College of Criminal Justice in New York City and a post-graduate certificate in Trauma Studies from New York University. She is also in her final year of a four-year certification in Core Energetics, a body-centered psychotherapy. Her psychotherapy practice focuses on trauma treatment, and how emotional and energetic issues manifest in the body.

Her inspiration for writing this book came from her love of massage and experience as a mother caring for her newborn daughter.

Joanne lives with her husband, Tim; her daughter, Ava; and her dog-daughter, Dakota, in Brookhaven, New York. She loves yoga and skiing and grudgingly practices Pilates. She can be reached at jbgshw@optonline.net.

Ilene S. Fox, LMT is a New York State Licensed Massage Therapist. She graduated from the New Center for Wholistic Health, Education and Research in 1998. She holds certifications as an Infant Massage Instructor and in Pre/Post Natal Massage. In addition to her private massage practice, Ilene is employed at the State University of New York at Stony Brook as a massage therapist in the Department of Pediatrics/Division of Infectious Disease. Here she teaches infant massage instruction to caretakers of HIV-exposed newborns and provides massage therapy to HIV/AIDS-infected children, adolescents, and young adults.

Ilene wanted to write this book because she believes massage therapy adds peace and calm to a world of chaos. Creating a book that teaches parents to massage their babies can only make the world a better place.

Ilene loves music, travel, yoga, and, of course, massage. She lives on Long Island and can be reached at peacepipe62@hotmail.com.

Dedication

From Joanne: For Ava — this book is so much about you.

From Ilene: To all of the babies and the people who care for them.

Contents at a Glance

Introduction...1

Part I: Nothing Quite Like Touch 5
Chapter 1: Welcoming Your Baby into the
   Wonderful World of Massage...7
Chapter 2: Understanding the Benefits of Baby Massage 19
Chapter 3: Getting to Know Your Baby Better 31
Chapter 4: Preparing for the Big Massage...45

Part II: Different Strokes for Different Folks:
Massaging Baby 61
Chapter 5: Massaging the Front Side 63
Chapter 6: Massaging the Face and Neck..87
Chapter 7: Massaging the Back Side 107

Part III: Making Massage Part
of Your Baby's Life..129
Chapter 8: Preemies and Newborns..131
Chapter 9: Older Babies and Toddlers 145
Chapter 10: Fitting Massage into Nap, Bath, and Diaper Time.........159

Part IV: Easing Health Problems
with Massage 177
Chapter 11: Massage for Common Ailments and Problems.............179
Chapter 12: Massage for Emotional and Developmental Issues.......199
Chapter 13: Massage for High Risk Babies 219

Part V: The Part of Tens....................................239
Chapter 14: (Almost) Ten Special Techniques 241
Chapter 15: Ten Great Massage Resources..247

Index 251

Table of Contents

Introduction 1

About This Book 1
How To Use this Book 2
How this Book Is Organized..................................2
    Part I: Nothing Quite Like Touch 2
    Part II: Different Strokes for Different Folks:
      Massaging Baby 2
    Part III: Making Massage Part of Your Baby's Life 3
    Part IV: Easing Health Problems with Massage 3
    Part V: The Part of Tens....................................3
Icons Used in this Book...3

Part 1: Nothing Quite Like Touch........................5

Chapter 1: Welcoming Your Baby into the Wonderful World of Massage 7

Focusing on Quality, Not Quantity...........................7
Recognizing the Need for Touch..............................8
    Considering our changing values 8
    Choosing attachment parenting 9
    Spoiling your baby?......................................10
Massaging Your Baby from Head to Toe 11
    Using Swedish massage techniques.................11
    Acing Massage 101......................................13
    Benefiting all ages: Preemies to toddlers 14
    Healing and tending to special needs 16

Chapter 2: Understanding the Benefits of Baby Massage 19

Bonding with Your Baby: It's a Good Thing!..............19
    Getting in touch 19
    Releasing a bonding hormone 20
    Promoting trust...20
    Communicating...21
Becoming a More Confident Parent.........................21
Managing Stress 22
    Taking Stress 101 23
    Realizing the serious effects of stress...............24
    Identifying signs of stress..............................24
    Keeping your own stress level in check 25
Aiding with Postpartum Depression 26

Promoting Growth, Development, and Overall Health 27
    Stimulating your little one..27
    Encouraging weight gain...28
    Helping with digestion 28
    Enhancing neurological development................................28
    Bringing on sensory awareness..29
    Strengthening the immune system....................................29
    Providing self-soothing skills 30

Chapter 3: Getting to Know Your Baby Better 31

Tuning In to Your Newborn's Needs.....................................31
    It's gonna be alright: Comforting your little one 32
    Easy does it: Calming the jumpy baby.......................34
    The power of touch: Responding to your
        baby's need for contact 35
Getting Into a Routine (6 Weeks to 3 Months) 36
    I'm talking to you! Understanding
        your baby's cries..37
    It's playtime: Encouraging joy, pleasure, and fun.......38
Changing from Caterpillar to Butterfly (3 to 6 Months).......38
    Making friends..38
    What's next? Relieving boredom 39
    Getting a workout 40
    Drooling, sucking, crying . . . I'm teething! 40
Becoming an Individual (6 Months to 1 Year)......................41
    Look out! Gaining mobility 41
    Understanding separation anxiety:
        It's a two-way street...42

Chapter 4: Preparing for the Big Massage........... 45

Good Vibrations: Getting in the Mood to Massage...............45
    Identifying readiness cues...46
    Clarifying your intentions..46
    Moving slowly and smoothly 46
    Breathing properly: The relaxation response.............47
    Having good posture 48
Finding the Right Time to Massage 49
Finding the Right Place for Massage 49
Massaging Safely 50
Selecting an Oil to Use..50
Setting the Tone 51
    Playing music 51
    Singing favorite songs 52
    Using aromatherapy..53
Knowing When Not to Massage 54
    Using abdominal massage wisely 54
    Overstimulation: Following your baby's cues............54
    When in doubt, leave it out: Using your
        common sense 55

Trying Out Your First Massage..............................55
Setting the scene.......................................55
Applying the oil..56
Practicing your technique: The Dolphin Stroke 56

Part II: Different Strokes for Different Folks: Massaging Baby..................................*61*

Chapter 5: Massaging the Front Side 63

Soothing the Feet and Legs...................................63
The Taffy Pull 64
Kneading Dough...65
Squeeze and Twist 66
Thumb Circles 67
Ankles Away 68
This Little Piggy 69
Raking...70
Combining strokes......................................71
Relaxing the Belly 72
The Water Wheel..72
Thumbs to Sides 73
Sun and Moon 74
I Love You 75
Opening the Chest and Shoulders 76
The Heart Stroke.......................................77
The Open Book Stroke 78
The Butterfly Stroke 79
Reaching for Arms and Hands..............................81
Alternating Hands 81
The "C" Stroke...81
Wrist work 83
Hands on hands 83

Chapter 6: Massaging the Face and Neck 87

Proceeding with Caution...................................87
Soothing Your Baby's Smile 88
Relaxing the jaw 88
Loving those sweet cheeks: The Smile Stroke 91
Relaxing the Eyes 93
Smoothing Out the Forehead 94
The Open Book Stroke 94
Big Circles 96
The Temple Stroke......................................99
Paying the Ears, Chin, and Neck Some Attention 101
The Ear Stroke...101
Chinny Chin Chin 102
Working the neck 104

Chapter 7: Massaging the Back Side 107

Taking Advantage of Tummy Time 107
Massaging the Legs and Feet...108
  The Taffy Pull 110
  Kneading Dough...110
  Thumb Circles..110
  Ankles Away 112
Bottoms Up! Kneading Your Baby's Bottom 112
  Alternating Thumbs 112
  Circular Palmer 113
  The Large Bottom Stroke 114
  Finger stroking 115
Doing the Back Stroke 116
  The Long Effleurage Stroke 118
  Back and Forth...119
  Swooping 121
  Small Circles..122
  Sacral stroke..124
  Raking..125
Relaxing the Neck and Shoulders: Long Strokes.................126

**Part III: Making Massage Part
of Your Baby's Life 129**

Chapter 8: Preemies and Newborns 131

Handling an Early Arrival...131
  Finding time for touch in the hospital 133
  Continuing contact when you get home...................136
Welcoming Your Newborn Bundle of Joy............................138
  Providing contact through clothing...........................140
  Establishing a massage routine at home 140
  Using touch while you nurse your baby...................141
Adding to Your Massage Routine..................................143

Chapter 9: Older Babies and Toddlers 145

Holding Still: Keeping Your Child's Interest.....................145
  Massaging your older baby 146
  Massaging your toddler 148
Making Massage a Family Affair 150
  Including your older child 151
  Getting creative with family massages 152
Using Massage to Your Toddler's Advantage.....................152
  Setting and respecting boundaries...........................154
  Teaching discipline through massage.......................155
  Handling tantrums...156

Chapter 10: Fitting Massage into Nap, Bath, and Diaper Time 159

Choosing the Right Time..159
Deciding Whether to Stimulate or Not 160
    Very young babies 160
    More experienced babies 161
Massaging Baby Before or After Nap.......................161
    Knowing how much sleep to expect 162
    Realizing the importance of naps 162
    Timing your massage right.....................................163
    Giving a great massage before a nap......................163
    Giving a great massage after a nap.........................165
    Waking your baby gently with massage....................168
Taking Baby in the Bath with You 168
    Playing it safe 169
    Bathing with a newborn..169
    Giving your newborn an after-bath massage 171
    Bathing with your older baby 171
    Giving your older baby an after-bath massage.........172
Bringing Massage to the Changing Table..................172
    Changing your newborn 172
    Changing your older baby 174
Making Daily Massage Routine................................174
    Creating rituals...174
    Giving a five-minute massage................................175
Identifying More Good Times and Places for Massage 176

Part IV: Easing Health Problems with Massage 177

Chapter 11: Massage for Common Ailments and Problems 179

Relieving Constipation 179
    Bypassing the problem with breastfeeding..............180
    Recognizing discomfort in formula-fed babies 180
    Saving solids until baby is ready 180
    Counteracting constipation...................................181
Recognizing and Responding to Colic......................181
    Looking for causes of colic....................................182
    Massaging to ease colic 182
    Offering your baby additional relief 183
    Easing your own stress 184
Breathing Easy: Coping with Asthma 184
    Reducing asthma triggers.....................................185
    Seeing signs of asthma...185
    Recognizing asthma attacks..................................186
    Massaging for asthma 186

Ouch! Helping Teething Pain 186
    Anticipating their arrival 187
    Recognizing signs of teething.......................187
    Massaging to ease the pain 188
    Offering additional relief................................189
Alleviating Chest and Sinus Congestion.................189
    Knowing the difference: Cold versus flu....189
    Massaging to ease chest congestion 190
    Massaging to ease sinus congestion 191
    Minimizing your baby's risk 191
Helping Your Fussy Baby 192
    Identifying fussy factors 192
    Offering comfort through touch and massage..........193
    Dealing with high need babies 194
Healing Your Baby's Skin..196
    Treating eczema...196
    Caring for cradle cap.......................................197

Chapter 12: Massage for Emotional and Developmental Issues 199

Overcoming Attachment Issues 199
    Recognizing patterns of attachment 200
    Bonding with an adopted or foster child.....201
    Dealing with Reactive Attachment Disorder 205
Coping with Developmental Delays 206
    Identifying causes of developmental delays 206
    Realizing effects on attachment....................207
    Trusting the benefits of touch and massage...........207
    Working with muscle tone 208
Handling Special Needs and Siblings.......................216
    Being honest..216
    Minimizing rivalry...217

Chapter 13: Massage for High Risk Babies 219

Babies Born to Addiction..219
    Helping the drug-addicted baby 219
    Addressing fetal alcohol syndrome................223
Babies Exposed to HIV 228
    Navigating pregnancy with HIV.....................228
    Massaging babies with (or exposed to) HIV 232
    Using other complementary therapies.....................234
    Taking universal precautions 234
Additional Resources 235
    For babies affected by drug and
       alcohol addiction 235
    For babies and children affected
       by HIV and AIDS...237

Part V: The Part of Tens......................239

Chapter 14: (Almost) Ten Special Techniques.......241

Trying Massages from Other Parts of the World 241
  Indian massage...241
  Tui Na massage 242
  Shiatsu massage..243
  African massage..243
Stretching...243
  Arm stretches..243
  Leg stretches 244
Helping Your Baby's Posture 245
  Supported sitting......................................245
  Unsupported sitting 246
Bringing Baby into Your Yoga Routine 246

Chapter 15: Ten Great Massage Resources.........247

Surfing the Web 247
  www.InfantMassage.com 247
  www.AskDrSears.com 248
  www.HealthyFamily.org..................................248
  www.LittleForest.com 248
Finding Massage Associations 248
  American Massage Therapy Association 248
  International Association of Infant Massage............249
  International Loving Touch Foundation 249
  Associated Bodywork & Massage Professionals 249
Using Videos 249
  Baby Massage and Exercise 249
  Infant Massage/Postnatal Yoga Combo Pack 250
  Exercise with Daddy & Me..............................250

Index 251

Introduction

The fact that you've picked up this book and are reading this page tells us that, most likely, you've heard of baby massage. You may not know why or how to do it, but you're curious to find out. That's great: That's what we're here for!

If, on the other hand, you picked up this book because you had some time to kill browsing in the bookstore and never realized that such a thing as baby massage existed, that's fine, too. We're an equal opportunity informer, and we welcome you to our pages.

In case you need convincing that this book is worth taking home, consider this: Baby massage is a practice that has been around for centuries, and recent research indicates that it provides both emotional and physical benefits for your little one (and a wonderful opportunity to increase the bond between the two of you).

We save the details for the chapters that follow, but before we get to the meat and potatoes of baby massage, we need to explain a bit about how we put this book together.

About This Book

Our goal with this book is to enhance a wonderful longstanding tradition with contemporary knowledge — essentially, to fuse the past and the present. (How's that for a tall order?) We want to help you, as a parent or caregiver, realize that you have the ability to positively influence your baby's health and that the steps to accomplishing that aren't very complicated. Our hope is that we can encourage you to make massage part of your everyday relationship with your baby so you can reap the many benefits.

You'll notice that throughout the book, we tie together the technical aspects of massage — the specific hand positions and strokes you use — with both medical and philosophical reasons for doing them. But don't let a little philosophy make you nervous; we don't expect you to automatically feel comfortable with every idea we present. Our purpose is to offer a holistic approach to massage so you can decide what works for you and your baby.

How To Use this Book

Like every *For Dummies* book, this is a reference book. No, that doesn't mean it's like an encyclopedia; it means that we don't expect you to read it from cover to cover. (Of course, if you find it so compelling that you can't miss a single word, we won't complain!) This book is designed so you can pick and choose which chapters you really want to focus on, and within each chapter you can find all the information you need to understand that particular subject.

You'll notice that we include lots of artwork in this book. That's because we realize you may have an easier time understanding what we're saying if you can see examples. But while the photos and illustrations are a great complement to the text, they can't substitute for the step-by-step instructions for each massage technique. We encourage you to use the words and images together to perfect each technique.

How this Book Is Organized

This book is divided into the following five parts.

Part I: Nothing Quite Like Touch

In this part, we share with you all the wonderful reasons to massage your baby. We detail the benefits for you, the parent or caregiver, as well as for your baby. You discover how your baby's development is influenced by touch, as well as the steps you can take to prepare for giving your first massage.

Part II: Different Strokes for Different Folks: Massaging Baby

In this section, we show you the actual techniques for massaging your baby. We cover all parts of your little one's body, from head to toe, front to back. What works for some babies won't work for others, so we offer a smorgasbord from which to choose so you can find out what techniques work best for you and your baby.

Part III: Making Massage Part of Your Baby's Life

Babies change so dramatically during their first years that we can't simply assume that the massage your baby enjoys at 3 months will still satisfy her at 2 years. And babies who are born early have special needs and limitations. In this part, you find in-depth information about massaging your preterm baby, as well as your older baby or toddler. We also discuss how you can work massage into your everyday life.

Part IV: Easing Health Problems with Massage

One of the great benefits of baby massage is that it can help alleviate many common health problems, from constipation to teething pain. It can also have positive effects on emotional issues and reduce stress and encourage development in babies with high-risk issues, such as fetal alcohol syndrome and drug addiction. We cover each of these topics in this part.

Part V: The Part of Tens

Each *For Dummies* book has a Part of Tens, and this is no exception. This last part offers you quick information on different massage and stretch techniques to add to your repertoire, as well as massage resources, including Web sites, national organizations, and videos.

Icons Used in this Book

As you read, you'll notice little circular works of art in the margins. These are the book's *icons*, and here is what they mean:

We get a little philosophical from time to time. This icon lets you know that a bit of wisdom from Eastern philosophies or *energy medicine* — a belief that your body is made up of different systems of energy that need to be balanced to promote health — is nearby.

Some bits of information are worth tucking into your mental file cabinet for future reference. The job of this icon is to alert you that such useful information is nearby.

We try not to get too technical in this book, but we also realize that some people like to know details about why something works, as well as how. If we're going to throw clinical jargon or heavy ideas your way, this icon warns you that they're coming.

When you see this icon, you'll know that the paragraph it accompanies contains ideas that can make massaging your baby as easy as possible.

Every once in a while, we need to alert you to reasons why you shouldn't perform a certain massage technique or the potential for causing your baby harm. That's the job of this icon.

Part I
Nothing Quite Like Touch

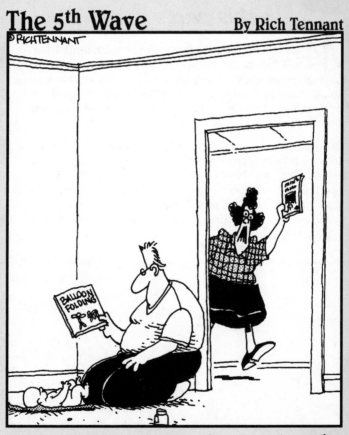

The 5th Wave   By Rich Tennant

"Mike! Wait! I gave you the wrong book!"

In this part . . .

Massaging your baby involves so much more than just technique. In this part, we show you what baby massage is all about. There are plenty of wonderful reasons to massage and touch your baby. We make sure you are versed in the benefits of baby massage for both you and your baby.

You also get an idea of how you can incorporate touch into your baby's growing emotional and developmental needs. Plus, we show you everything you need to get started with baby massage, from oils and music to timing, good posture, proper breathing, and right intention. And we give you an easy practice massage to try. You're well on your way!

Chapter 1

Welcoming Your Baby into the Wonderful World of Massage

In This Chapter

▶ Realizing the importance of attachment

▶ Getting a brief introduction to massage technique

▶ Anticipating the benefits of massaging your baby

*Y*ou have so many good reasons to massage your baby, and this chapter introduces you to the biggies. We discuss how and why you can use massage as a tool to foster and enhance your attachment with your baby. We also touch on the physical benefits of baby massage — including how you can use massage to help treat and prevent certain illnesses.

Along the way, we introduce you to the basics of Swedish massage — the foundation of the techniques we demonstrate in later chapters. And we explain how you can adapt your massage routine to accommodate the needs of babies at different ages and stages of development.

Focusing on Quality, Not Quantity

If you recently became a parent, you may have spent the last nine months preparing for birth and connecting emotionally with your baby. Or maybe your pregnancy was unplanned and your experience has been laced with anxiety and self-doubt. Perhaps infertility plagued your attempts to get pregnant, and now your dreams of parenthood are finally realized, either through birth or adoption.

Regardless of how your baby came into your life, or what your parenting circumstances are, baby massage is a great way to create a relationship with your little one. Spending even five minutes massaging your baby each day creates a space for bonding and relaxation for both of you that can stay in your baby's memory for a lifetime.

We have all heard that the quality of time we spend with our children — not the quantity — makes a difference. There is no greater manifestation of this truth, no better example or opportunity, than to give love to your child through massage. Time spent massaging your baby involves genuine, undivided attention that is experienced as love and pleasure. Intend your massage as a gift, and it will be received as such.

Recognizing the Need for Touch

In other cultures — which some people might label primitive — mothers typically carry their babies with them all the time. These mothers are very attuned to their babies' needs and respond to them quickly and naturally with ease. This bonding approach to parenting breeds intuition and compassion, and it begins with touch.

Considering our changing values

Before the inventions of anesthesia and baby formula, all mothers felt the birth of their children and the sensation of their children suckling on the breast. Since these inventions, values have changed in our culture, as have conventional wisdoms.

The choices many parents now make when giving birth are based on cost- and time-effectiveness — if not for the parents themselves, at least for the hospital and its staff. Nature's primal callings have been minimized by a healthcare profession that has to manage huge demands on its time. *Epidurals* (a form of anesthesia delivered through the spine) are the norm, and Caesarean deliveries are performed in as many as a quarter of all pregnancies. During much of the twentieth century, formula was touted as the best option for mother and baby; breastfeeding was considered an inferior feeding method and an inconvenience.

We certainly understand that sometimes Caesareans and epidurals are medically necessary, and some of the changes that have occurred have resulted in greater health for mothers and babies.

However, we also recognize another result of our changing values: Opportunities for touch and bonding between parent and child have been reduced.

Another factor that impedes the bond between parent and child is a detached approach to parenting, which nurtures laziness or apathy. Parents are only human, and the demands of everyday life, particularly with an infant or young child, are enormous. *Detachment parenting* is an invitation to do and care less. We all have within us the capacity to be lazy or believe we deserve a break. That's why it's important to consciously make a commitment to attachment-focused nurturing and bonding. If you invest energy today, you will reap rewards throughout your life.

Choosing attachment parenting

So what exactly does the term *attachment parenting* mean? Attachment parenting is a philosophy of parenting that emphasizes creating a secure attachment with your baby. Just about all the advice we give in this book is aimed at encouraging attachment parenting. This parenting style is about being sensitive to your children, getting to know them and their needs, and relying on your own intuition as a parent.

Using the right tools

While there aren't any specific rules or guidelines to follow to practice attachment parenting, here are some tools you can use that make a secure attachment with your child more likely:

- ✔ Massage your baby.
- ✔ Breastfeed.
- ✔ Avoid separations.
- ✔ Co-sleep (see Chapter 3).
- ✔ Wear your baby in a sling (see the sidebar "The art of baby wearing" later in this chapter).
- ✔ Bond with your baby immediately after birth (see Chapter 3).
- ✔ Respond to your baby's cries.
- ✔ Feed your baby on cue, not on a schedule.

Not all these tools will work for you, your baby, or your family. That's why relying on your intuition is so important. You can formula-feed your baby and sleep in separate rooms and still be practicing attachment parenting.

Seeing the benefits

To many people, the term *attachment parenting* probably sounds scary. After all, we want our children to grow up and be independent, not attached to our hips for the rest of our lives, right?

A better term to describe this parenting style would probably be *healthy interdependent promoting parenting.* But that's just too much of a mouthful.

Whatever you want to name it, this approach to parenting has many benefits:

✔ Your baby learns to trust you.

✔ Your baby grows into a sensitive and empathic child and adult.

✔ Your baby learns *interdependence:* how to care about and connect with others in a compassionate and cooperative way.

✔ Because attachment-parented babies spend less time crying than others, their energy goes into growing and learning. Attachment-parented babies also tend to be more alert and focused.

✔ Attachment-parented babies are more confident.

✔ You become more sensitive.

✔ A deep attachment between you and your baby is formed.

✔ You have a happy baby whose needs are met and feelings are respected.

Spoiling your baby?

New parents sometimes hear advice from older generations — and child development experts — about not spoiling their children by giving them too much attention and responding immediately to their needs. Theories about child development have changed radically through the years. Not long ago, new parents were advised to ignore their babies' cries to be fed in order to create a strict feeding schedule. And recently, sleep trainers have become popular, helping new parents get their babies onto a sleep schedule as early as possible.

While these practices serve a purpose — creating predictable routines early in an infant's life — they can contribute to a sense of separation between parent and child. This is just one more reason to make a conscious choice to devote time to bonding through touch and massage.

Bringing infant massage to the Western world

The founder of the International Association of Infant Massage, Vimala McClure, discovered infant massage during her travels in India in the early 1970s. In Indian culture, the mother massages everyone in the family and passes the tradition down through her daughters. McClure found that massaging babies was a wonderful way to soothe and communicate nonverbally with them. When McClure contracted malaria, all the local women massaged and sang to her. The feeling in her body resulting from the massage stayed in her memory.

What McClure experienced in India simply didn't exist in Western culture at the time. She wrote *Infant Massage* in 1979 to remind us that love, security, and compassion are a type of wealth. She created the International Association of Infant Massage to offer opportunities for this type of touch to anyone. Infant massage instruction now takes place all over the world. We want to acknowledge and thank Vimala McClure for bringing infant massage to our attention. Her work reminded us of what we once knew but learned to forget.

In Vimala McClure's book *Infant Massage,* she writes, "As with fruit, neglect rather than attention spoils a child." You are the center of your baby's world (and she is the center of yours!). Your baby relies on you for everything: food, love, safety, nurturing. We believe that if *spoiling* refers to giving your baby lots of love and attention and responding to her needs, then by all means, you should spoil away!

Massaging Your Baby from Head to Toe

The techniques we show you in this book fit under the category of *Swedish massage.* They have been adapted to be useful for babies and toddlers.

Using Swedish massage techniques

The origins of Swedish massage can be traced to Per Henrik Ling (1776–1839), the "Father of Massage," who cured himself of rheumatism with a brand of massage that he called *medical gymnastics.* Today, a Swedish massage performed on an adult consists of specific strokes done in the following order:

1. **Effleurage.** These gliding strokes can be deep or superficial and help to warm the superficial muscles.

2. **Petrissage.** These strokes reach the deeper layers of muscle tissue by lifting the muscle.

3. **Friction.** By working with the fibers of the muscle, friction releases any scar tissue that may restrict movement.

4. **Tapotement.** These strokes include tapping or hacking the muscles and can either stimulate or sedate depending upon the rhythm and pressure used.

5. **Vibration.** This technique involves shaking or rocking the muscles to induce either a stimulating or sedating effect on the body.

6. **Joint motion.** Putting a joint through its complete range of motion helps alleviate any restrictions in movement.

With babies, you don't need to use all the strokes of Swedish massage, and you may move the order of the strokes around. Slow, rhythmic strokes are the most soothing to a baby. For a very young

Researching the benefits of touch

The Touch Research Institute (TRI), located at the University of Miami School of Medicine, was founded in 1992 by Tiffany Field, Ph.D. TRI conducts research on the effects of touch and works to apply these findings to science and medicine.

Here are some of TRI's findings:

✔ Newborns who are exposed to cocaine in utero gain weight faster and show less signs of stress if they are massaged.

✔ Fathers who massage their babies for 15 minutes daily experience more favorable interactions with their infants.

✔ Depressed mothers touch their babies differently than mothers who aren't depressed, which can negatively affect growth patterns in newborns. Research studies show that if depressed mothers massage their infants, the babies gain weight more quickly, have more organized sleep/wake behaviors, are less fussy, are more sociable and easily soothed, have better interaction behaviors, and have lower levels of stress hormones.

✔ Premature babies receive the most significant benefits from massage. These infants gain more weight, sleep better, and are discharged from the hospital sooner if they receive massage.

✔ Newborns exposed to HIV gain more weight if they receive massage.

infant, holding and rocking (a form of vibration) may be enough. Being present and aware of your baby's responses and needs will guide you in your choice of strokes.

Some strokes, if performed too vigorously, can be harmful to a baby; for example, you never want to use deep friction or heavy tapotement on an infant.

Any kind of contact with your infant — even just having him near your body — is the basis for beginning to massage your infant. As your baby gets older and more used to massage, he can tolerate more strokes, and you will be able to massage your baby from head to toe.

Acing Massage 101

The goal of Swedish massage is to increase the circulation of blood and lymph fluids in the body. The fluids are pushed out of the muscle tissue, back into the circulatory system, and out of the body through the elimination process.

Toxic material (in the form of lactic acid) accumulates in our bodies — specifically in our muscle tissues — as a result of poor diet, overmedication, exercise, illness, or dehydration. This toxic material results in knots, *trigger points* (tender, painful spots located on a very tight muscle), *adhesions* (areas where muscle and fascia — which we define in a moment — adhere to one another), and scar tissue. These problems cause pain, discomfort, and restriction of movement. Injury and poor posture can put muscle tissue into spasm to protect the area from further harm, causing patterns of pain.

Massage therapy works the soft tissues of the body so they can function optimally. Massage therapy is the only form of bodywork that addresses the soft tissue specifically, putting the body back into *homeostasis* (balance).

Consider this analogy: Think of the body as a sweater. If you pull one corner of the sweater, it changes the shape of the entire sweater. Massage puts the soft tissue — your sweater — back into its proper shape.

The body is lined with *fascia,* which is like a netting that holds everything in place. Keeping the integrity of the fascia is one of the main goals of massage therapy. Injury, adhesions, scar tissue, illness, disease, and spasms all pull on the fascia, resulting in stretching the sweater out of shape.

Prenatal massage

Pregnant women experience extreme changes in their bodies. Prenatal massage is a great way to alleviate some of the discomforts caused by pregnancy, such as sciatica, joint pain, fatigue, hormonal imbalances, edema, leg cramps, and constipation.

Make sure that your massage therapist has training in prenatal massage, because she needs to be aware of some things to avoid. For example, it is not safe to massage the belly during the first trimester. In addition, some points in AMMA (an Asian type of massage) can trigger a miscarriage. As long as your massage therapist is properly trained, massage during pregnancy is perfectly safe.

An added bonus of prenatal massage is being able to lie on your belly. Some massage therapists use a special type of cushion (placed on top of the massage table), which can allow you to safely lie on your belly even in the third trimester!

Your coauthor Joanne highly recommends receiving regular prenatal massages: During my recent pregnancy, I had weekly massages and found that the more I relaxed, the more relaxed my baby became. After Ava was born, I used a stroke on her belly that was similar to the stroke used on my abdomen. She loved the stroke, and I believe it was familiar to her. She melted like butter on the changing table!

Benefiting all ages: Preemies to toddlers

Baby massage is a wonderful form of touch for babies of all ages. Even babies in utero can benefit from massage (see the sidebar on "Prenatal massage").

Preparing yourself mentally

No matter how old your baby is, be genuine, present, and attentive with him. Massaging your baby without intention is, frankly, a waste of time. Intention is simple, but it requires sincerity, focus, and presence. You can establish intention by saying something like, "I am here for you my little one, to love you, to care for you, to make you feel comfort and love." Be sure you are fully present as you say the words; infuse them with feeling and sincerity.

Most of us don't realize how often we detach ourselves from the world. While we sit in the presence of others, we spend a lot of time drifting off or becoming distracted. This is so common it is regarded as normal. Unfortunately, our interaction with others suffers silently; our connections are compromised.

You will find this to be true when you are challenged to stay 100 percent present with your baby during massage. Breathe deeply, powerfully, and steadily, and project love toward and into your baby as you massage her. Keep your entire attention focused on your presence and interaction with your baby. This is a challenge, but it is completely within your capability. With practice, you will quickly become more aware, more regular in your breathing, and more focused.

Working with a premature baby

A study conducted by Touch Research Institute in 1986 showed that premature infants who receive some kind of touch in the hospital gain up to 47 percent more weight than those who don't. The sooner premature babies gain weight, the sooner they are able to come home.

If you have a premature baby, all you need to do to bring massage into his life is to touch him with your finger. Believe it or not, just the touch of your finger stimulates his growth and development.

Being touched increases circulation in any area on your baby's body. Increased circulation is physically stimulating, as well as encouraging to overall growth and good health. Gentle massage is a basic and loving method to help your preemie along. It is also a great way to bring physical connection into your baby's world. Watch your baby react in wonder and pleasure, and you'll know you're on the right track.

The art of baby wearing

You have probably seen other moms and dads carrying their babies around in slings. Wearing your baby in a sling offers a feeling of comfort and safety similar to what is experienced in the womb.

Let's be blunt: Being born is stressful. Labor can be difficult, everything is new, and babies have to learn how to get their needs met. Wearing your baby provides her the comfort of motion and close contact with you. It also strengthens bonding. You can begin to use a sling with your newborn right away. It's an easy and convenient way to nurture your baby while you do errands or just move about your house. (Your coauthor Joanne wrote many pages of this book wearing her baby in a sling!) Wearing your baby is also an easy way to be sure that your baby has all the touch and contact she needs as a newborn. Baby wearing can be likened to a hands-free massage!

Massaging newborns and infants

Holding, rocking, and gently stroking are usually enough to create an attachment and calm and soothe your newborn baby. If your baby is crying, remember to maintain a deep, self-nurturing, steady breathing. This prevents you from becoming stressed and over-whelmed, which makes it easier for your baby to relax.

As your baby grows older and is able to tolerate more touch and stimulation, you will be able to use the massage techniques we show you later in the book (see Chapters 5, 6, and 7). Even if you have just started to massage your infant, have fun, and don't be afraid to experiment!

Touching your toddler

When your baby is no longer a baby, you can add more strokes to your repertoire depending on your baby's attention and tolerance level. If you have been massaging your toddler since infancy, you will know her needs for touch very well by this point. You can increase the length and frequency of your sessions. Don't be surprised when she begins to ask you for a massage!

If you haven't been massaging your young one up to this point, it's not too late to begin. In Chapter 9, we offer all sorts of tips to help you keep your mobile 1- or 2-year-old interested long enough for you to massage her.

It's also not too late for your toddler to reap the benefits of baby massage. You can use this time to strengthen your bond, teach her how to relax, and soothe her hardworking muscles!

Healing and tending to special needs

Baby massage is a great holistic tool to use — always in conjunction with medical advice, of course — to help your baby with common ailments and different developmental needs.

Some massage techniques are effective when medicine isn't. Anyone with a colicky baby will attest to the fact that they would do any-thing to stop their baby from being in pain, and to stop the crying. A simple belly massage may feel good to your baby and ease the pain. Obviously, massage isn't a substitute for professional medical care, but offering massage is a conservative way to begin treating common ailments.

Offering preventative medicine

Massage is a great way of preventing your baby from becoming sick or stressed by maintaining his health. Regular massage keeps the body in *homeostasis* (balance) by increasing circulation, improving the efficiency of the elimination process, relieving stress, and improving immune function. Massage is a simple and effective way of preventing illness.

Treating physical problems

In Chapter 11, we focus on common ailments or physical problems that massage can help alleviate. Massage can be an effective treatment for the following problems common to babies:

- ✔ Slow weight gain
- ✔ Teething
- ✔ Colic
- ✔ Sleep problems
- ✔ Stress
- ✔ Digestive troubles
- ✔ Chest and sinus congestion

Easing emotional stress

As we discuss in Chapter 12, massage can also help babies deal with emotional issues, such as the following:

- ✔ Attachment/bonding
- ✔ Socializing
- ✔ Relaxation

Having faith

Faith is an elusive quality. We invite you to have faith in massage as an approach to healing, as well as in your ability to administer it. Your baby can and will enjoy your loving touch, and using this opportunity to heal and help your loved one is a powerful and empowering experience.

In the United States, we tend to turn to doctors, hospitals, and the pharmaceutical industry for health and healing. But for centuries, the Asian cultures (particularly the Chinese) have relied rather successfully on holistic, hands-on healing practices. Massage is both a medical and a holistic treatment.

Unleashing endorphins

Endorphins are our bodies' natural painkillers. A release of endorphins (commonly referred to as a *runner's high*) leaves you feeling euphoric instead of fatigued, over-worked, or exhausted. The deep relaxed state that massage induces triggers the release of endorphins. Keep this in mind when your baby is teething or stressed from colic. With massage, you can treat the cause of the pain and its symptoms, plus you can provide your baby with a natural, drug-free painkiller.

Chapter 2

Understanding the Benefits of Baby Massage

In This Chapter

▶ Bonding with your baby

▶ Increasing your confidence as a parent

▶ Reducing your baby's stress level (and your own)

▶ Dealing with postpartum depression

▶ Encouraging your baby's health and development

*B*aby massage isn't just something that you do *to* your baby; it's a way of communicating through touch how much love you have for your little one. Massage offers almost as many benefits to you, the caregiver, as it does to your baby. This chapter explains the many wonderful reasons to bring massage into your baby's life, from promoting a positive bond to reducing your baby's stress.

Bonding with Your Baby: It's a Good Thing!

Many new parents, upon arriving home with their babies, are in awe of the responsibility of parenthood and — to be perfectly honest — terrified by it. If you know many couples who have had children, chances are you've heard at least a few of them admit to looking at each other after their homecoming and saying, "Now what?"

Getting in touch

A hospital is not always an ideal setting for beginning the bonding process with your newborn. Even if you had zero opportunity to bond with your baby in the hospital, you can start doing so as soon as you get home, and touch — including massage — is the ideal way to begin.

All you really need to do to begin bonding is to touch your baby a lot. Hold him, rock him, wear him in a sling, or sway with him every chance you get. Bonding can occur during feeding, changing, and sleeping, as well as during times when you're massaging your little one. Young babies aren't frequently alert and attentive, but luckily you don't have to wait for these times to promote bonding. Your intention, and how much energy you are willing to direct toward your baby, are the key factors.

Bonding with your baby creates a secure and healthy attachment between you two. Your baby internalizes this feeling of safety, which leads to him being easier to comfort and more affectionate.

Releasing a bonding hormone

The bonding benefits of touch and massage aren't strictly emotional. There is a physical basis for the connection that develops between mothers and babies during massage.

Massage stimulates the release of oxytocin in a mother's body. *Oxytocin* is a hormone that serves some key functions during and after pregnancy. For example:

- Oxytocin stimulates the mother's uterus to contract during labor.

- Oxytocin promotes the *let-down reflex* during breastfeeding — the reflex that moves milk into the breast so the baby gets food when he sucks.

- Oxytocin is continually released whenever a mother nurses, and it helps to relax the mother and nurture the bond between mother and baby during breastfeeding.

When a mother massages her baby, she stimulates the release of oxytocin in her own body, which facilitates attachment and bonding. Through physical touch, she promotes a deeper emotional connection with her infant.

Promoting trust

Babies need a *lot* of touch and holding. The best advice we can offer new parents is to approach each day of parenting with a clear understanding of how important touch is — especially in the first six weeks to two months of life, when many babies need constant holding or touch during their awake time.

With that said, you want to also realize that touch and holding are only part of the picture — the physical part. If you touch your baby frequently but do so without paying any attention to what you're doing, you (and your baby) aren't reaping the full benefits of the contact. You must also be attuned to your baby. By *attuned* we mean being as present as possible whenever you hold, touch, and carry her. Doing so will satisfy her need for comfort and safety more fully than touch alone.

Through her earliest interactions with you, your infant discovers what it means to count on other people — to trust. Babies who are massaged tend to develop strong feelings of trust for their caregivers, and as a result they also tend to have experiences with other people that are warm, nurturing, and loving. Your first experiences in touching your baby are essential in creating a trusting relationship between the two of you. These early moments truly lay the foundation for your relationship.

Communicating

As we all know, communication can take many forms; we pick up messages in a variety of ways, not all of them verbal. When you massage your baby, you and your baby have many opportunities to express yourselves nonverbally.

Here are just two examples of nonverbal communication that can be expressed during a massage:

✔ Babies learn to see themselves through their caregivers' eyes. Providing eye contact during a massage gives your baby the opportunity to feel loved and to have his sweetness and vulnerability mirrored back to him through your eyes.

✔ When you massage your fussy baby, you model relaxation with your relaxed and soothing touch.

During massage, your baby picks up cues from you. Don't underestimate how much information your baby absorbs through observation. Babies are like sponges, absorbing everything within reach.

Becoming a More Confident Parent

Lots of parents are unsure about what to do with a baby; if you're anxious about your perceived lack of parental skills, you have lots of company. Baby massage offers parents an easy way to have nurturing, loving contact with their babies.

Spending quality time with your baby gives you the chance to figure out his cues. You discover things like:

✔ His likes and dislikes

✔ Good (and not-so-good) times for massages

✔ Indications that he is tired or hungry

✔ Meanings behind his expressions

The more you know your baby, the easier it becomes for you to respond to his needs, which in turn gives you more confidence as a parent.

No matter how many books you read or how many other parents you talk to, you're bound to have insecurities when you become a parent. Touching your baby is a basic, primal, and effective way to build a positive relationship. Throughout infancy and into childhood, most young ones want and need to be touched frequently. Massage is simply a systematic approach to satisfying your child's basic needs.

Keep in mind that massage isn't just for moms and babies. Fathers sometimes feel left out during a baby's early years, especially if the baby is being breastfed. If you're a new dad, you may assume that your baby's needs are being met already and you don't have much to contribute. But your baby needs your touch, too! Baby massage gives dads — as well as other caregivers — an opportunity for bonding and intimacy that is all their own. If you work full-time and don't always feel like a vital part of the parenting team, baby massage gives you the opportunity to spend irreplaceable quality time with your baby.

Managing Stress

Stress is what we all experience when we are faced with challenges or feelings that we find potentially overwhelming. Stress can be created by either positive or negative situations. Think about planning a wedding and filing for divorce. Although one situation is assumed to be positive and the other negative, both situations create a lot of stress. Many causes of stress are unforeseeable; we can't possibly predict everything that can bring stress into our own lives, let alone the lives of our babies.

Are you surprised that babies experience stress? Consider that infants experience new feelings and situations every day — many of which create excitement, joy, and wonder, but others of which aren't quite so pleasant. Babies also feel stress when they have colic, are teething, or have a depressed caregiver.

Babies' bodies accumulate stress, just like yours and mine. Identifying your baby's stress cues and responding to them with massage are effective ways to help her relax and let go of that accumulated stress.

Taking Stress 101

Stress is the culprit behind most of the illnesses and issues that baby massage helps to alleviate and prevent. At the risk of getting a little technical, we thought you'd like to understand why that's the case.

The autonomic nervous system

The stress response is regulated by the autonomic nervous system (ANS), which consists of two separate systems:

✔ **The sympathetic nervous system:** When we experience a threat, the sympathetic nervous system is engaged by the release of the stress hormones adrenaline and cortisol (which we explain in the next section). Our heart rate and blood pressure increase, our muscles become contracted, and we are on alert. The sympathetic nervous system is concerned with activities that expend energy stored in the body.

✔ **The parasympathetic nervous system:** The parasympathetic nervous system kicks in when the threat is gone. The job of this system is to conserve energy to allow for relaxation. Our heart rate and blood pressure decrease, and our muscles begin to relax. Through relaxation, this system increases the energy stored in the body.

Stress hormones

There are two major stress hormones: *adrenaline,* which puts you on alert for danger, and *cortisol,* which provides you with energy to take on the threat.

During stress, adrenaline is secreted through the adrenal gland and is responsible for increasing our heart beat and blood pressure, among other things. The release of adrenaline activates the famous *fight or flight* response, and we are on the lookout to either stand our ground or run away from danger.

In order to create more energy so we can handle the next stressful situation, our adrenal gland also secretes cortisol. The secretion of cortisol triggers the release of amino acids, which raises our blood sugar level in order to have more glucose for energy. The excess energy created is our way of physically trying to handle stress.

Realizing the serious effects of stress

Stress wreaks havoc on both adults' and babies' bodies. The effects of stress can include physical problems, such as chronic illnesses, as well as emotional difficulties, such as attachment issues. We discuss these issues (and how to use massage to alleviate them) in Part IV of this book.

While you can't possibly remove all stress from your baby's life, you can help to manage and alleviate stress through touch and massage. Massaging your baby activates the parasympathetic nervous system to bring on relaxation and lowers the levels of stress hormones in your baby's body.

Identifying signs of stress

Now that you understand why your baby experiences stress and the reasons you want to help her deal with it, how do you know when it's happening? Following are some typical signs that your baby is stressed:

- ✔ **A heightened startle response:** It's normal for babies to have a startle response; reacting to new noises or experiences shows that the nervous system is working. You'll know that your baby's startle response is heightened or exaggerated if she is jumpy or reacts in fear to noises or situations that are familiar to her.

- ✔ **Fussing/complaining:** Babies can fuss for a lot of reasons. However, if your baby is cranky and whiny in addition to showing some of the other indications we list here, she may be stressed.

- ✔ **Crying:** Babies have different kinds of cries to alert their parents that they are hungry, bored, tired, or hurt. Stressed babies are difficult to soothe immediately; they continue to cry and fuss even when held.

- ✔ **An arched back:** Squirming and arching the back (like a cat) are signs of stress.

 ✔ **An increased breathing rate:** Babies have tiny lungs. Prolonged crying increases their breathing rate, and stress increases their heart rate.

 ✔ **Shaking/twitching:** If your baby is shaking or twitching, chances are that she is frightened. We suggest that you hold her for comfort to calm her down before giving a massage.

If you see that your baby is stressed, gentle strokes used in a downward direction (like the Dolphin Stroke we present in Chapter 4) can help your baby learn to relax.

The effects of massage are cumulative: The more your baby receives massage, the easier time she'll have being able to relax. After she receives consistent, regular massage, your baby will remember and look forward to your cues for relaxation: the feel of the oil, the sound of soft music, the sound of your breath, and the feel of your hand on her body. She'll also start to remember what it feels like to be relaxed, helping to ensure that she can relax herself in between sessions.

Keeping your own stress level in check

Babies are very sensitive to energy. Your own emotional state and level of relaxation affect how your baby feels. To massage your baby effectively, with the goal of reducing his stress, you must take the time to breathe and relax before you begin.

Have you noticed that when you feel stress, you hold your breath? Holding your breath is a common way to avoid feeling something uncomfortable or painful.

The simplicity of touch relaxation

One of the best ways to help your baby cope with stress is also the easiest. To trigger feelings of safety and warmth, gently and securely hold your baby — help her feel as if she were still in the womb. Look into her eyes and tell her something like, "It's okay, I understand how hard it is to be a baby. I'm here with you, and you can relax now."

Use this touch relaxation technique anytime: during a massage; while bathing, holding, or rocking your baby; while the baby is in a sling; during a diaper change; or whenever you sense that your baby is becoming overstimulated.

Following is a simple exercise in diaphragmatic breathing for you to use just before you massage your baby, or anytime you feel stressed:

1. **Place one hand on your lower belly, and the other on your chest.**

2. **Breathe in through your nose, and imagine your belly is a balloon that you are filling with air.** Notice with your hand that your belly rises before your chest.

3. **Let the breath move up from your belly into your chest.**

4. **Feel the breath move up from your chest to your throat.**

5. **Exhale through your nose.**

6. **Repeat as necessary.**

Diaphragmatic breathing is the way that babies breathe naturally — until they experience stress, that is, and learn to hold their breath to avoid feeling. This breathing exercise elicits relaxation by engaging the parasympathetic nervous system, which we explain in the "Taking Stress 101" section earlier in the chapter.

Another technique you can use to reduce your own stress is called the *relaxation response.* This meditation asks you to focus on a certain word or phrase in order to take your mind off the stress you're experiencing. In Chapter 4, we walk you through this meditation step-by-step.

Aiding with Postpartum Depression

Lots of women experience mood changes, anxiety, difficulty focusing, and increased sensitivity after giving birth. These emotional changes, which usually go away within a few weeks of birth, are typically signs of the baby blues and are not necessarily cause for concern.

Postpartum depression, however, is a much more serious matter. The onset of postpartum depression is usually caused by a combination of hormonal changes, sleep deprivation, change in lifestyle, and a sense of being overwhelmed with parental responsibilities.

The symptoms of postpartum depression are similar to the symptoms of major depression; the defining difference is that the onset of symptoms of postpartum depression occurs within four weeks of giving birth. Following are symptoms of major depression:

 ✔ Feeling depressed and crying a lot

 ✔ Losing or gaining weight

> ✔ Lacking interest or pleasure in the baby or other activities
>
> ✔ Experiencing insomnia or, conversely, sleeping more than usual
>
> ✔ Feeling suicidal and/or having thoughts about death or hurting the baby
>
> ✔ Having very little energy
>
> ✔ Having difficulty focusing

Mothers who have postpartum depression typically do not touch their babies often. Subsequently, the mother/infant interaction is minimal and lacks nurturing and warmth.

If a mother with postpartum depression can consciously create a time and space to touch her baby through the use of massage, the bond between mother and child is strengthened, and the infant begins to respond to his mother with warmth and pleasure. Being on the receiving end of a baby's love helps depressed mothers begin to feel the joy that is part of motherhood. That joy, in turn, can help to reduce the symptoms of depression.

If you know a mother with postpartum depression, help her initiate contact and touch with her baby. The symptoms of the depression make it next to impossible for her to attempt to touch or massage her baby on her own. However, with the help of a partner or family member, she can create a daily routine for touch and massage. It's important for the partner or family member to play a supportive role and to let the mother actually massage the baby.

Promoting Growth, Development, and Overall Health

Massaging your baby on a regular basis encourages alertness, increases weight gain, aids in digestion and neurological develop-ment, and increases sensory awareness. That's quite a package!

Stimulating your little one

Even with so much to see and do that is completely new, babies can get bored. Massage increases circulation, enhances you baby's alertness, and provides a new learning experience. Massage gives babies an opportunity to discover the different parts of their bodies, as well as to explore their feelings. Massage promotes an appropriate level of arousal for babies; they learn to be more attentive and less distracted.

In Chapter 4, we show you how to keep your baby's interest and stimulate him with music and singing during your massage.

Encouraging weight gain

When gauging a newborn baby's health, one of the first signs doctors look for is weight gain. If you want to impress your doctor with how fast your little one can gain weight, incorporate a 5- to 15-minute massage into your daily routine. Massage relaxes your baby and aids in digestion (which we discuss next), so food is better absorbed. Better absorption gives your baby a better than average chance of gaining weight.

In addition, massage stimulates growth-enhancing hormones. Have you ever wondered why animals lick their young just after birth? Touch is nature's way of stimulating growth. Remember this every time your dog starts to lick you and won't stop: Your pet is just responding to his intuition. (Maybe he thinks you could stand to gain a few pounds!)

Helping with digestion

Massage stimulates the digestive system. When anyone (including a baby) is under stress, the sympathetic nervous system shunts blood away from the belly to the larger muscles. The lack of blood and oxygen in that area shuts down the digestive system in order to provide energy elsewhere in the body.

The increased circulation that massage provides in the abdomen brings blood and oxygen to the intestines, which improves your baby's ability to digest and eliminate food.

Your digestive system works like a muscle. The smooth muscles contract to push food down through the esophagus to the stomach and out of the body through elimination. Massage encourages *peristalsis* — the pushing out of food stuffs in an orderly way through smooth muscle contractions.

Enhancing neurological development

Massage enhances your baby's brain growth. Studies have shown that massaging your baby speeds nerve *myelinization* — the growth of the fatty insulating material that encloses certain nerve fibers. When this insulating material — the *myelin sheath* — appears, nerve impulses can travel at a faster rate.

> # Getting defensive
>
> In Chinese medicine, the body's immune system is called *Wei Chi,* and it is created by the lungs and kidneys. This system is our natural defense mechanism. Imagine Wei Chi as a fence around you; if there is a hole in the fence, what is threatening you can get in. When your body is weakened and fatigued, your Wei Chi becomes vulnerable and can no longer protect you effectively. Disease and illness can enter your system. In Chinese massage and acupuncture, the Wei Chi is strengthened by balancing the lung and kidney energy, which protects you from becoming ill.

How does a speedy nerve myelinization translate into enhanced development in your baby? Look for some of the following signs:

✔ An ability to stay focused and alert for reasonably long periods of time

✔ Enhanced curiosity

✔ Strong memory skills

✔ Accelerated developmental skills

Bringing on sensory awareness

Massage enhances body awareness — it helps babies become more knowledgeable about their bodies in relation to the world. For example, babies discover their range of motion — what their limits are and what they can do. Massage also teaches them about having or experiencing pleasure in their bodies.

Strengthening the immune system

You may have noticed that you become more vulnerable to illness during stressful times. The same is true for babies. Massage increases the immune function by strengthening the relaxation response and decreasing stress hormones.

Because massage also aids the effectiveness and efficiency of other body functions (such as the circulatory and elimination systems), massage can strengthen your baby's body to fight off illness. In addition, massage increases your baby's lymphatic flow, which strengthens her body's ability to fight infection.

Making your child more resilient to stress

Following are some ways you can begin increasing your child's resiliency to stress as early as infancy:

✔ Create a relationship with your baby that promotes trust. You can do this by taking your child's needs seriously and responding to them in a timely manner.

✔ Have empathy and compassion for your baby, especially when your baby is crying or has colic. Being on the receiving end of empathy encourages your baby to feel empathy for others and compassion for herself.

✔ Keep in mind that your baby takes in everything that you do and learns from your actions. Be a role model in handling stressful situations.

Providing self-soothing skills

Thumb-sucking, rocking, and carrying a blanket or stuffed animal are ways that babies and toddlers soothe themselves. Adding massage to your baby's experience provides another self-soothing skill. The ability to calm himself down and deal with his emotions will help your child well into adulthood. Self-soothing skills help children become more resilient: Your child will be better able to handle and recover from stressful situations.

Massage helps your baby calm himself down by teaching him what it feels like to relax. The more frequently your baby experiences relaxation in his body, the easier it becomes for him to bring his body back into a relaxed state on his own.

 Simply holding your baby teaches him valuable self-soothing skills. The more frequently your baby experiences feeling safe and secure, the easier it is for him to create these feelings for himself as he gets older.

Chapter 3

Getting to Know Your Baby Better

In This Chapter

▶ Anticipating your baby's emotional development

▶ Understanding the need for touch at every age

▶ Using massage to meet your baby's needs

*W*hether your baby is a newborn or heading into the toddler years, her emotional needs are essentially the same: She needs to feel loved and secure. But as she grows and changes, the means of providing her that love and security can grow and change as well.

Massage is a great tool for helping you meet your baby's emotional needs at every stage. In this chapter, we show you how to combine knowledge of your baby's emotional development with knowledge of her desire for touch so you can meet her changing needs.

Keep in mind that we don't go into a lot of detail in this chapter about your baby's development; we hit the highlights so you can start thinking about how massage can work at any stage of infancy. If you're looking for more specifics about what to expect from your baby at any given age, check out *Parenting For Dummies* by Sandra Harding Gookin and Dan Gookin (Wiley).

Tuning In to Your Newborn's Needs

If you are like many parents, you have prepared for your baby's arrival by decorating the nursery, deciding whether to use a crib or co-sleep, and securing the infant seat in your car. You have researched breastfeeding versus using formula, completed your childbirth education classes, and are practicing your labor breathing techniques. You have done everything you can think of to prepare for the birth of your baby and welcome him home. What's left?

Thanks to years of research on child development, you have the opportunity to know and anticipate what your baby's needs are going to be. This means you can consider how you will be best able to fulfill them before you even get home from the hospital.

Most information about child development tends to focus on what a baby should be able to do by a certain age. This information is important, because it indicates how well your baby is developing and alerts you to potential developmental problems that need attention. However, equally important is information about babies' emotional development, and this information isn't always as readily available. In the following sections, we discuss both types of development.

How you handle your baby's emotional needs helps determine how easily your baby handles life's stresses, especially in regards to relationships. You are your baby's role model for how relationships should be.

It's gonna be alright: Comforting your little one

When babies come into the world, they have little awareness of you, their selves, and their surroundings. Their task is to become accustomed to life outside of the womb. Your job is to make this process a gradual one. Here are a few things to do that can make your job easier:

- ✔ **Get attuned:** *Attunement* literally means tuning in to your baby's energy and emotions — having a rapport with your baby. If you're lucky, you and your baby are a good fit from the beginning: For example, you want to hold and comfort your baby as much as she wants you to.

    Parents who do not have such an easy fit need to make extra efforts to see the problem, understand it, and make changes to fit their baby's needs. For example, if your baby doesn't like to be held a lot, and you want to hold him day and night, try not to take it personally. Your baby is not rejecting you; in fact, he literally doesn't know that you exist as a separate person yet! It's just that his needs for touch may be different than yours.

- ✔ **Reduce stimulation:** Fortunately, most babies are born with a "stimulus barrier" that screens out distractions and protects them from becoming overstimulated. For example, on the day your coauthor Joanne and her husband brought their daughter home from the hospital, they set the car alarm off while she was inside, buckled in the car seat. She didn't even flinch, nor did she seem to notice the noise. (Of course, we were horrified at our mistake!)

As babies' nervous systems develop, they are able to take in and handle more and more distractions and noises. Until then, and at least for the first six weeks or so, your job is to keep the stimulation level low. However, keep in mind that the womb is a very noisy place, so you don't need to maintain silence around your baby. Just be mindful of a lot of distractions that could be overstimulating.

If you have toddlers or other older children around, make them aware of the need to keep the noise level a little lower than normal, for example. Soon enough, your baby will come to enjoy their antics, and you will find yourself thanking them for distracting and stimulating your little one!

✔ **Be prepared for a lack of schedule:** Very young babies tend to get their days and nights mixed up, plus they need to feed every two to four hours (depending on if you are breastfeeding or using formula). The first six weeks or so can be a nightmare for any parent. Have patience: Remind yourself that your baby isn't behaving this way to make your life hard; she's just figuring things out. Remember that this is just a period of development, and things will change. It won't always be this hard!

Your baby has a job to do

According to experts in infant development, babies have certain tasks to complete in each stage of life before they move on to the next. If the baby doesn't achieve a task (such as learning to trust, for example), that may be an issue throughout childhood and into adulthood. For your baby to move on to toddlerhood, he needs to complete the following tasks:

✔ Learn to trust

✔ Learn to feel good about himself

✔ Manage the stress from different developmental stages (such as handling separation from you)

✔ Become aware of his body and begin to use it

✔ Express his emotions

Bonding in a hospital bed

Chances are that your experience with delivering a baby in a hospital will be much different than the experience your mother had. For example, most hospitals today are sensitive to the effects of lighting and noise on newborns. In many labor and delivery rooms, you find soft lighting and nurses speaking quietly. The reason for this is we want to welcome babies into the world with warmth and sensitivity. Emerging into this world can be shocking and sometimes even traumatic, and harsh lights and loud voices certainly don't help.

Another significant change is that most hospitals and birthing centers now encourage bonding through touch right away. Rather than a newborn being taken immediately to the hospital nursery, in many cases the baby is placed on the mother's chest just after birth. Also, new parents are encouraged to share a room with their newborn. Keeping your baby at your side during the hospital stay, rather than in the nursery (which is sometimes located on a separate floor!), promotes bonding by giving you more opportunities to touch and hold your baby.

You can definitely use massage as a way to attune with your baby and sensitively manage his stimulation level. Unfortunately, massage can't help you get your baby onto a feeding and sleeping schedule any sooner. However, Chapter 2 offers suggestions for relaxing and breathing through stressful times when you are feeling overwhelmed and sleep-deprived.

Easy does it: Calming the jumpy baby

If you're one of the lucky parents whose baby was easy from the beginning, count your blessings! If not, and your baby screamed constantly from the minute you arrived home, she needs extra care and sensitivity. Following are some suggestions to help:

✓ **Wrap your baby in a burrito.** Very nervous babies like to be swaddled, because it reminds them of the womb. Swaddling is an effective way of giving your baby the sensation of being held. Jumpy babies have frequent startle responses: Your baby's arms and legs will flail about, which scares her even more. She isn't even sure about having her own body at this age, and all that uncontrollable movement can be frightening.

Here is how to swaddle your newborn:

• Lay out a thin cotton or flannel receiving blanket.

• Fold the top right corner about 6 inches.

- Place your baby on her back in the center of the blanket with her head above the fold.

- Pull the right bottom corner across her body and tuck the edge under her back on her left side.

- Fold the bottom corner up (under her chin, if you need to).

- Bring the left corner over your baby's right arm and tuck it under her back on the right side.

Some babies don't like their arms tucked in, so you can just leave their arms free.

✔ **Get support.** High need babies are super sensitive. If your baby is jumpy from birth, screams a lot, needs to be fed every hour, and seems to rarely sleep, you may have a high need baby. If so, you have our understanding, and you will probably need a lot of support. Check out *The Fussy Baby Book: Parenting Your High-Need Child from Birth to Age Five* by William and Martha Sears for strategies and survival tips. You can also find lots of helpful information on their Web site: www.askdrsears.com. Good luck!

Because jumpy and high need babies are so sensitive, it's a good idea to keep your massages gentle and soothing. In Chapter 8, we give you suggestions for how to give a massage and prevent overstimulation.

The power of touch: Responding to your baby's need for contact

In the first month of life, your baby needs to be held a lot. Feeling safe and secure in your arms keeps him warm and gives him the gradual adjustment to life outside the womb that he needs. If you find the constant holding difficult to manage, invest in a sling (see Chapter 1) and carry your baby around.

We think it's a great idea for you to introduce massage to your baby at this young age. However, you must keep the following in mind: Babies feel vulnerable (and cold!) without their clothes on. You may want to try the massage techniques we show in Chapters 5, 6, and 7 with your baby's clothes on. Your baby will still enjoy the contact and reap lots of benefits from it. But he will also feel secure, and you are less likely to overstimulate him.

Considering co-sleeping

Under the right conditions, *co-sleeping* — sleeping in the same bed with your baby — is not only safe but can actually reduce the risk of sudden infant death syndrome (SIDS) and crib-related accidents.

If you decide to share your bed with your baby, keep in mind that research has shown mothers tend to demonstrate more protective behaviors toward their babies than fathers do during the night. In other words, it's often best if a mother sleeps next to her baby because mothers tend to be more aware (even in their sleep) of their babies' movements.

Here are some more safety tips to make co-sleeping work for you:

✔ Use a firm mattress, and don't use a fluffy comforter or pillows.

✔ Never, ever smoke in bed.

✔ Do not sleep with your baby if you use sleeping medication or are under the influence of drugs or alcohol.

✔ Do not sleep with your baby if you are sleep-deprived.

✔ If you want to co-sleep but are uncomfortable sleeping with your infant in bed with you, purchase a co-sleeper or three-sided crib that can act as a sidecar.

✔ Use guardrails on your bed, and/or place your mattress on the floor.

There are many benefits to sleeping in the same bed with your baby. For one, if you are a nursing mother, you will get more sleep (a big plus) because you won't have to get up to breastfeed. Here are some others:

✔ Your breathing regulates your baby's breathing. Because your baby hears you breathe, it reminds him to breathe (which helps reduce the risk of SIDS). Plus, babies spend less time in deep sleep when they co-sleep due to mom's movements during the night. (Deep sleep can be dangerous for babies at risk for SIDS.)

✔ Babies sleep better, too. Because they do not have to cry to get their mothers' attention for feedings, they don't fully wake up, and they fall back asleep faster.

✔ Co-sleeping fosters attachment (which we discuss in Chapter 1).

✔ Your baby continues to receive comfort and nurturing from you throughout the night.

Getting Into a Routine (6 Weeks to 3 Months)

When your baby passes the six-week mark, you should notice that life starts getting a little easier. Your baby should begin making patterns in behavior that start to look like a routine.

This is a good time to start incorporating massage into your baby's routine. Experiment and find a time that works for both of you. For example, your coauthor Joanne found that during the first three months of giving her daughter massages, the massages' effect was very energizing. For that reason, it was better to schedule massage time early in the day. Your baby, however, may enjoy a massage before a nap if the massage helps him to sleep.

If you're reading this section while tending to the needs of a brand new baby, you may be wondering how you'll ever know when "before a nap" is? If your baby is like most, at this age she will probably sleep about 16 hours a day (although not in one chunk of time!). You will notice that sleeping tends to occur after a feeding, so as you get into a more predictable feeding routine, you should be able to better anticipate her sleeping schedule as well.

One problem that you may experience during this time period is the dreaded colic. Colic typically runs its course between the age of 6 weeks and 3 months. In Chapter 11, we provide you with information about colic and some massage techniques that can help to alleviate the discomfort.

I'm talking to you! Understanding your baby's cries

Babies cry because they need something, and this is the only way they can get your attention. At this age, babies do not have the cognitive development or ability to manipulate. They depend on you responding to their cries so they can get their needs met.

You may notice that your baby's cries seem to be different now than during the first few weeks of life. Early on, you probably felt the demand and desperation in her cries. Now that you have been responding to her needs, she is beginning to learn to wait for you to respond, as she expects her needs to be satisfied. Her cries usually start to sound more like requests.

At this age most babies' cries usually mean that they are:

- Hungry
- Tired
- Bored
- Needing to be held
- Overstimulated

At this age, a baby's cries usually stop when you pick her up and hold her.

It's playtime: Encouraging joy, pleasure, and fun

Your baby is just beginning to notice that he has a body (although he isn't yet aware that his body is separate from yours). His hands start to open and grasp for things (like your hair!). You can encourage body exploration and fun by making massage part of your playtime. Begin by naming body parts as you massage them: "This isn't a turkey drumstick — it's your leg!" You and your partner may be the only two to get the joke, but your baby will pick up on your enthusiasm and enjoy it.

Your baby is also beginning to learn the difference between pleasure and pain. Yet, he hasn't completely figured out that you are typically the cause of both. (Nursing brings pleasure; 2 a.m. diaper changes in February bring, if not pain, at least discomfort.)

At around the age of 3 months, your baby's smile response peaks, and you will feel rewarded for all the hard work and love you have given your baby.

Changing from Caterpillar to Butterfly (3 to 6 Months)

At this age your baby is becoming increasingly sociable. Her sensory awareness has increased, so she has discovered her body and is aware of the world around her. She gurgles, screeches, babbles, and coos. You no longer have a little newborn around the house, but a new member of the family!

Making friends

In an attempt to stimulate their babies, many parents spend a lot of time and money shopping for toys developed to raise their child's IQ or teach babies how to perform a specific task.

The most important kind of stimulation your baby can receive involves people and relationships. In fact, the kind of relationships she has and what she learns from them (such as trust versus mistrust) establish the foundation of her future personality.

If your social butterfly is bored and craving contact, give her a massage! She'll appreciate the social contact, and you don't have to buy another toy to provide the stimulation she needs.

Secure babies love to meet other people and are especially fascinated by other children. However, they are also becoming pickier about who they socialize with. Don't worry, your baby isn't becoming a snob; instead, she's in the early stages of *separation individuation.* What does this mean? At around 6 months of age, you will notice your baby becoming more active and wanting to explore all kinds of new stuff. In psychology, we call this *hatching.* This means your baby is getting ready to see new things and separate from you — not physically, mind you, but your baby is in the very early stages of realizing that she is a separate person.

What's next? Relieving boredom

Babies need to play. Play activities help to stimulate and rescue them from long, boring days of nursing and sleeping.

You may find your baby's demands for stimulation exhausting, but remember: At this age her needs and wants are the same. Your baby does not know how to ask for something that is more than she needs.

At this age, your baby is stimulated by objects that are slightly different than those she is familiar with (such as a teething ring of a different color than her other ones). Introducing something new and unfamiliar is fairly easy to accomplish.

From 3 to 6 months, babies are fascinated by people's faces. They love to watch people's expressions and body language. Your baby is beginning to notice that there is a world outside of her relationship with you.

Good enough parenting

Thankfully, you don't have to be perfect to be a good parent. You just have to be "good enough." In fact, it's good for both you and your partner to provide just enough frustration for your baby to learn that he has to ask for what he needs, and that all his needs are not going to be met.

But you don't have to force the matter, either. Try not to create situations where your baby's needs won't be met; these situations occur naturally. For example, your baby may need to be held *now!* but you are stuck in rush hour traffic and can't pull over. You can try to soothe him by talking to him, but he will have to wait and bear the frustration of not being held when he needs to. You will probably feel guilty or pained by his frustration, but keep in mind that you are helping him grow and tolerate frustration by being nurturing and sensitive.

As part of this early stage of separation, you may notice that as you hold your baby, she pulls back to scan your face and grab onto your hair (quite hard, unfortunately!) or even your earrings if you wear them. Your baby is checking to see how you and she are different from one another.

You can use massage to satisfy a couple of needs. Massage gives you and your baby something to do each day, and you can vary the techniques you use in order to keep her interest. Plus, you can give your baby a massage on the front side (see Chapter 5), which affords her plenty of "face time" while protecting your hair and jewelry!

Getting a workout

Now that your baby has discovered her body, she is also figuring out that she has some control over her movements. Gone are the days that your little munchkin bounces all over the place without control. Now she is able to see an object, recognize it as something familiar, and grasp it. This may seem simple to you, but to a baby, hand–eye coordination is huge!

You probably can't remember having the ability to put your big toe in your mouth, nor can you imagine how much pleasure this activity involves, but your baby will remind you!

All this grasping, batting, kicking, and attempting to roll over can wear a baby out and create physical stress. Your baby needs your help to release any tension and stress from her body with a daily massage.

Drooling, sucking, crying. . . I'm teething!

Somewhere between the age of 4 months and 2 years, most babies begin to teethe. How will you know when it starts? Your baby will have a constant need to suck on something, produce lots of drool (enough to soak a bib), and possibly cry out in pain unexpectedly.

When teething starts, a parent's first response is to want to do something — anything — to alleviate the baby's obvious discomfort. Want some great news? You can use massage to soothe away your baby's stress from teething. In Chapter 11 we explain techniques you can use to help your baby endure teething discomforts.

Becoming an Individual (6 Months to 1 Year)

The second half of a baby's first year is action-packed. And even as your baby grows into a little person who can crawl, explore, and maybe even walk on his own, the opportunities for massage continue — as long as you make the effort to keep up!

Look out! Gaining mobility

By 6 months, most babies have the neuromuscular control to be able to get into a sitting position by themselves. However, balancing their bodies in a sitting position is still an issue, so many topple over until they gain full control. Around the same time that they are perfecting sitting up, babies begin to practice crawling.

Babies vary greatly in their development during this age range: Some babies begin to pull themselves up and stand before they even begin to crawl. At almost 6 months, your coauthor Joanne's daughter crawled on her back by arching her back, lifting her pelvis, and propelling herself across the floor. Babies thoroughly enjoy the newfound freedom of movement!

Person permanence

Your baby is not able to hold a mental image of you in her mind until around 12 to 18 months. Until that age range, babies are not cognitively able to understand that you exist if they can't see you.

Keep this in mind when your child is experiencing separation anxiety. What triggers the anxiety is a lack of understanding why or where you have gone, which creates a feeling of loss for babies who are not yet autonomous (independent) at this stage. It's not that your baby thinks you won't come back when you leave for a while; she simply doesn't have the ability to put together the concept that you will be back later.

Every time that you leave and come back reinforces person permanence. Your baby will not be completely comfortable being separate from you until age 3, which is when most children begin nursery school.

Your baby's new ability to control her body means that most likely she will become more interested in moving around and exploring the environment than being held. This fact may lead you to believe that your days of bonding through massage are over. Not true.

Mobile babies still need touch. They may not need to be held as much as newborns, but at this stage, their need for touch is about reconnection. Massage helps you let your baby know that you encourage her exploration, but you are still there to love and comfort her when she gets back.

 Create a ritual by massaging your baby at the same time daily or weekly. Your baby will look forward to the contact, which will make it easier for you to keep her still long enough to be massaged.

Understanding separation anxiety: It's a two-way street

One day you may try to drop off your 9-month-old at the babysitter's, and as you start to leave, your baby will turn to you, grab your leg, and start screaming. You'll probably feel terrible about leaving her, knowing that you have to go to work, and uncertain why she is so upset because she has never reacted this way before.

Unless your baby is having a premonition that you are about to leave her with the babysitter from hell, chances are that you and she are both experiencing separation anxiety. (See the sidebar "Person permanence" for more information about this normal developmental stage.)

Before the first episode of separation anxiety occurs, you may notice that your baby becomes more and more affectionate with you and begins to realize when you leave the room. These are signs that the separation process is beginning. Not until your baby experiences distress at your absence does it really become a problem for both of you.

 How you handle the separation can make all the difference in how your baby responds. Be sure to make all "bye-byes" feel positive to your baby by smiling and showing happy body language when you leave, not just when you come back.

If you need to leave your baby with a sitter, be sure to find a nurturing and warm caretaker who can best substitute for you in your absence. Don't switch sitters frequently; let your baby form an attachment with a consistent caretaker.

Securely attached babies sometimes have very strong reactions to separation. Very simply, these babies have learned that they feel good when they are with you, and they want those good feelings to continue!

Making massage routine after a separation gives you both a chance to reconnect and strengthen your attachment. (For more on attachment, see Chapter 12.)

Chapter 4

Preparing for the Big Massage

In This Chapter

▶ Making sure you're in the right mood

▶ Choosing a good time for the massage

▶ Getting the materials you need

▶ Recognizing when to avoid massage

Giving your baby a great massage involves more than using the techniques we show you in Part II of this book. It involves preparing yourself and your baby for the experience.

The timing of a massage matters, as does your mood. And although you don't have to buy a lot of fancy equipment to give a massage, you do want to make sure you have at hand everything to make the experience enjoyable for both of you.

In this chapter, we walk you through the things you need to consider before you schedule your first massage with your baby. We also help you get your feet wet by showing you a simple massage technique you can try your first time out.

Good Vibrations: Getting in the Mood to Massage

Have you noticed that whenever you are having a stressful day, your baby is too? That's because babies are very sensitive to our moods and energy. The best way to begin to prepare for giving your baby a massage is by being honest with yourself about whether the timing is right for you. If you know that you'll feel rushed, annoyed, or impatient, it's best for you and your baby that you skip the massage for now.

If, however, you want to try to improve your mood so you can give the massage despite the stresses you're feeling, using the suggestions in the following sections may help.

Identifying readiness cues

Before you work on getting yourself ready to offer a massage, try to determine if your baby is ready for one. How do you know? Later in the chapter, in the section "Knowing When Not to Massage," we discuss some specific situations when it's best to wait before massaging. But following are a few basic signs that indicate your baby is amenable to massage:

- ✔ She isn't fussy.
- ✔ She makes eye contact with you.
- ✔ She is interested in what you are doing — she's not trying to crawl away, roll over, or grab a nearby toy.

If your baby is distracted, you can certainly try to get her attention; the suggestions in Chapter 9 may help. However, if she doesn't seem ready for a massage and you aren't in a great mood either, it may be best to wait for a better time.

Clarifying your intentions

As we discuss in Chapter 2, there are lots of reasons to give your baby a massage. However, when you prepare to actually give a massage, it's best to push aside all those details about the benefits regarding health and bonding. Obviously, you'll keep the benefits in the back of your mind, but your goal should be to focus simply on the experience of sharing your love for your baby through touch.

Working from a place of kindness, compassion, and care is all you need to be able to give your baby a wonderful massage.

Moving slowly and smoothly

You want to move gently and slowly during your massage. Don't rush through the techniques we show you in upcoming chapters: Take the time to feel your baby's skin and let your baby feel and get used to your touch.

Be patient! Massage is a new experience for both of you. In the beginning, your baby may be able to tolerate only a few minutes of massage. This is perfectly normal because massage can be very stimulating. Try to avoid feeling like you have to complete a certain number of techniques in order for the massage to "count." It's fine to work only the baby's legs or arms, or even just his feet!

Your baby's tolerance level will increase with each massage. You will recognize that your baby's tolerance level is increasing by watching his body language. Notice how relaxed he is and whether he is making eye contact with you. (A tired or overstimulated baby may avoid eye contact.) Trust your instincts, and follow his cues.

How much pressure is too much for your baby? You want to use light to moderate pressure with a gentle touch. Think about turning an omelet: You need focus (so as not to break the egg), and you need to be decisive but careful. You will know when to increase the pressure of the massage by watching your baby's cues: His level of eye contact and relaxation are key.

You need to find the amount of pressure that's just right for your baby. If the pressure is too great, you'll know because it will leave red marks on your baby's skin. If you're not using enough pressure, you'll tickle your baby — the giggling will give it away!

Breathing properly: The relaxation response

In Chapter 2 we give you a simple instruction for diaphragmatic breathing that can help you relax in any situation, including before a massage. Here we want to share an exercise that can deepen your relaxation: the relaxation response.

Defined by Herbert Benson, MD, the relaxation response is a simple meditation designed to stimulate the parasympathetic nervous system — which we discuss in Chapter 2 — to evoke relaxation.

You can create the relaxation response by practicing the following exercise for 5 to 20 minutes per day. The more you practice relaxation, the easier it will be for you to relax into a deeper state in less time:

1. **Find a comfortable place to relax and close your eyes.**

2. **Begin diaphragmatic breathing (as we describe in Chapter 2 — see "Keeping your own stress level in check").**

3. **Progressively relax all the muscles in your body.** Begin with the top of your head, and imagine relaxation spreading down throughout your body, all the way down to your toes. Focus on each body part as you work your way down.

4. **To avoid letting any distracting thoughts enter your mind, begin to say (either silently or out loud) the word "One" on your out breath.**

   You may replace the word "One" with any other word or phrase that feels right. For example, you may say, "I am here" or "Relax."

We recommend that you use this technique on a regular basis. While it would be ideal to use it just before you massage your baby, we realize how impractical that could be. But if you can find the time to meditate regularly, your level of relaxation will increase, and all you will need to do before and during the massage is practice your diaphragmatic breathing (see Chapter 2).

Having good posture

No matter what your mother may have told you, having good posture means more than just sitting up straight! Good posture helps your breathing and level of relaxation. You can maintain good posture whether you are standing or sitting. The following tips should help:

- ✔ Keep your shoulders down away from your ears.

- ✔ Relax and soften your belly, but keep your spine long so you are not slouching.

- ✔ If you are standing, be sure to keep your feet parallel and your knees slightly bent. Make sure that you are not putting most of your weight on one leg, as doing so affects your posture.

- ✔ If you are sitting on the floor, you can sit cross-legged with your butt on the edge of a pillow. The pillow helps support you to keep your spine long with little effort.

Massage therapists learn to work from their *hara,* which is a Japanese word for "abdominal center." This area is the *solar plexus* — the energetic and physical center of your body. When you are breathing properly and working from your hara, you are able to move calmly, with confidence, and you are more likely to sense your own energy and the energy of your baby.

To get in touch with your hara, slightly pull your navel in toward your spine. Doing so, along with proper breathing, gives you the sensation of being in touch with the center of your body. You don't have to suck in your stomach (as if you were going to do a set of crunches) or scoop out your abdomen (as in Pilates).

Finding the Right Time to Massage

Choosing the right time to massage your baby is essential to achieving a good massage. Following are some guidelines to keep in mind:

- ✔ Avoid giving a massage immediately after your baby has eaten. Wait at least one hour before starting a massage.

- ✔ Try to work a massage into your daily schedule. Some of the best times to do so include:
    - Before or after a nap
    - Before or after a bath
    - After a diaper change

    We discuss nap, bath, and diaper time massages in detail in Chapter 10.

- ✔ Determine if your baby becomes stimulated or sedated during massage, and keep this in mind when choosing the time of day. You obviously don't want to massage a baby who becomes stimulated just before bed or nap time.

- ✔ Make sure that you have plenty of time to give the massage. If you're in a rush, your baby will sense your stress level, and the massage won't be as enjoyable or effective.

- ✔ Select a time of day when you won't be easily distracted, such as by other family members or other responsibilities.

- ✔ Find a time of day when you can turn the phone ringer off.

Finding the Right Place for Massage

The ideal place for you to massage your baby is where you both will be the most comfortable. The ideal place may depend on your baby's age and developmental skills. For example, your coauthor

Joanne massaged her daughter Ava on a bed until she began crawling. Now that Ava is on the go, the carpeted floor feels safer to me, because I don't have to worry about her falling off the bed. (Crawling babies are fast!)

Here are some suggestions for where to give a massage:

✔ On your bed

✔ On a carpeted floor

✔ On the changing table

✔ On a hard surface floor, using the pad from your changing table or some other cushioning material

✔ On your lap (see Chapter 7 for positions)

Massaging Safely

Obviously, you don't want to cause your baby any harm during a massage, and practicing safety is fairly simple. Here are some tips to follow before every massage:

✔ Wash your hands.

✔ Remove any rings or jewelry that may interfere with the massage or scratch your baby.

✔ Keep your nails filed.

✔ Make sure your baby isn't too hungry or too full. Either condition could cause him to spit up or even throw up.

✔ Pour the oil you will be using into a small bowl, and place it near your massage space. This way, you can quickly dip your fingers in and still maintain contact with your baby.

Selecting an Oil to Use

Skin is the largest organ in the body and can absorb toxins. For this reason, it's a good idea to use only natural products when massaging your baby. Following are examples of vegetable- or nut-based oils that are appropriate to use:

✔ Almond

✔ Grape seed

✔ Jojoba

> ✔ Olive
>
> ✔ Safflower

Your coauthor Ilene uses grape seed, almond, or jojoba oil. You can find these oils in supermarkets or natural food stores.

Because skin absorbs toxins, we do not recommend using baby oil or anything else made from petroleum products. If you can't eat it, don't use it!

If you are concerned about an allergic reaction to using a new oil (especially a nut-based oil), try a spot test. Massage oil onto a small patch of your baby's arm or leg. Wait 24 hours to see if any redness or other allergic reaction develops before using the oil on the rest of your baby's body.

See the section "Applying the oil" later in the chapter for instructions on how to put oils to use during a massage.

Setting the Tone

In this section, we show you some extras that you can include during your massage that help create the right mood for you and your baby.

Playing music

If you think that music will help relax you and your baby, consider before the massage begins what type of mood you're trying to create. For example:

✔ **Classical massage music:** What we're talking about here isn't necessarily Mozart or Bach. Instead, we're talking about standard massage music — music that is very relaxing and perfect for a serious massage. Your local music store probably carries CDs of massage music, which are usually located in the New Age Music section and typically have flute or harp instrumentals.

✔ **Fun massage music:** Instead of instrumentals and serious music, you may want to opt for lighthearted children's songs. You can find children's CDs at music stores and discount stores. Before you know it (and are ready to admit it!), you'll have all the words memorized and will be singing along to the CD, much to your baby's delight.

> ✔ **Calm lullaby massage music:** Playing lullabies is perfect if you're giving a massage before a nap or bedtime.

You can also purchase a sound machine that plays prerecorded white noise that simulates rain, ocean waves, a heartbeat, or even noises that babies hear in utero!

Singing favorite songs

If you're a great singer, your baby will love to hear your voice and will find it soothing and relaxing. And even if you're tone deaf or have a terrible singing voice, chances are your baby will still love to hear you sing. Your coauthor Joanne (who is terribly tone deaf) massages her daughter, Ava, while singing Ava's favorite song: Frère Jacques. (Yes, even babies can have a favorite song!)

As you're singing, feel free to get creative and to personalize the lyrics. For example, here are the traditional lyrics to Frère Jacques:

Frère Jacques (Brother John)

Frère Jacques, Frère Jacques,

Dormez vous? Dormez vous?

Sonnez les matines. sonnez les matines,

Din din don, din din don.

Your coauthor Joanne changes the lyrics for her daughter by singing:

Frère Jacques, Frère Jacques,

Dormez vous? Dormez vous?

Ava Amanda, Snowflake loves you,

We do too, we do too.

You may also incorporate nursery rhymes into your massage, which are especially entertaining to older babies and toddlers. We talk more about using rhymes during massage in Chapter 9.

You can find lyrics to many children's songs and nursery rhymes online at www.mamalisa.com. You can even create your own lullabies for your baby and have them recorded. You can find this service online as well at www.babybaby.com. The most important thing is to let yourself be creative and have fun.

Using aromatherapy

Aromatherapy uses *essential oils* to balance the mind, body, and spirit. How is an essential oil different from other oils? The essence of a plant is extracted and used to treat and prevent various diseases. There are literally hundreds of different types of oils (some of which are blends) that are used to treat illness. A commonly used essential oil is *tea tree oil,* which is often used to treat infections and to boost the immune system.

For adults, essential oils can be applied directly to the skin or heated in the room during a massage to release the scent. In our opinion, babies' skin is too sensitive to apply essential oils during a massage. However, if you want to use aromatherapy to enhance the atmosphere, we think that's fine.

We recommend that you wait until your baby is 6 months or older before you begin using aromatherapy. Essential oils contain powerful scents that may interfere with your baby's ability to recognize your scent.

If you would like to use aromatherapy during your massage, here are some tips to get you started:

- ✔ Invest in high quality oils, even though you will not be applying the oil to your baby's skin. We recommend Young Living Essential Oils; you can purchase them online at www.young living.us or look for them at natural food stores. These oils are made from high quality ingredients.

- ✔ Use a mild oil, such as lavender, which helps create a calm and relaxing atmosphere.

- ✔ Before you start your massage, take a trial run and test the amount of oil you're using. The aroma should not be overwhelming.

- ✔ Use a diffuser for the oils rather than a burner that relies on tea lights. A diffuser is safer because you don't have to worry about remembering to blow out a candle (losing your memory is part of being a parent!) or knocking the candle over. A diffuser releases oil slowly into the air by electrically heating a small plate where you place the oil.

  Electric diffusers range in price from about $20 to $120. You can find a nice selection at www.botanical.com.

Knowing When Not to Massage

Giving your baby a gentle, loving massage is never harmful (as long as you follow carefully the techniques we describe). However, at certain times that gentle, loving massage simply won't be received as well as at other times. In the sections that follow, we explain how to determine when it's best to set aside your massage plans until your baby is better prepared.

Using abdominal massage wisely

You want to use abdominal massage techniques carefully. If your baby is hungry when you try one of these techniques, she will probably become overstimulated or angry, and she (and you) will not enjoy the massage. On the flip side, if you massage your baby when she has just eaten, chances are she'll spit up or vomit. You must allow your baby at least one hour to digest whatever she has eaten before beginning the massage.

When you work on your baby's abdomen, always work in a clockwise direction. In Chapter 5, we give you the specifics of how to do so and why.

Overstimulation: Following your baby's cues

Your baby becomes overstimulated when he has had too much excitement from play, socializing, or other activity. When your baby is already overstimulated, you want to avoid massaging him until he's had a chance to calm down.

Following are some cues that your baby is overstimulated:

- ✔ He does not make eye contact with you; he may close his eyes or turn away.
- ✔ He fusses, whines, or cries.
- ✔ He arches his back.
- ✔ He tenses his body.
- ✔ He gets the hiccups.
- ✔ He yawns or falls asleep.

All babies have different stimulation levels. Baby massage helps to increase the amount of stimulation a baby can tolerate, and it helps parents become more sensitive to their baby's tolerated level of excitement.

When in doubt, leave it out: Using your common sense

If, at any time, you don't feel like a particular technique, stroke, or exercise is right for you or your baby, or if you are just unsure about doing it, we want you to skip it. Your baby certainly won't notice that you've left out a specific technique, but she will notice if your stress level rises during the massage because you're doing something that doesn't feel right.

When your baby has an injury of any kind, be especially careful to avoid any techniques that may aggravate it:

✔ Be sure to massage *around* — not over — any cuts, bruises, or rashes.

✔ Obviously, you also don't want to massage over a broken bone. Depending upon what bone is broken, you may want to avoid massaging the entire limb. If, for example, your baby has broken her wrist, you could leave the whole arm alone and massage the rest of her body.

In addition, do not massage your baby if she has a fever.

Massaging your baby fine-tunes the sensitivity you have as a parent, giving you more confidence and sharpening your instincts. In other words, it confirms your common sense.

Trying Out Your First Massage

In Part II of the book, we describe specific techniques for massaging each body part. But before we get there, we want to help you practice the steps you'll take to prepare for each massage you do.

Setting the scene

The first decision you need to make is whether to take off your baby's clothing, including his diaper. If you're massaging a very young infant, you may want to keep his clothes on so he doesn't become too stimulated.

If you remove your baby's clothing and diaper, lay your baby down on a couple of towels (in case of an accident!) on the changing table, the bed, or the floor. Have a clean diaper, wipes, and a fresh change of clothes nearby. Make sure your oil and a towel for your hands are within reach.

Check to be sure the room temperature is warm enough for your baby to be comfortable, especially if you're removing all his clothing.

Create a mood for the massage — perhaps by choosing music to play, plugging in an aromatherapy diffuser, and dimming the lights.

You may find that after you begin, your baby starts to fuss. Just follow his cues. If he's hungry, you may have to stop and feed him. If he's becoming overstimulated, take a deep breath, relax yourself, and stop the massage. Pick him up and gently hold him until he calms down.

Applying the oil

Following are the steps for applying oil that you can use before starting any massage:

1. **Place a small amount of oil (approximately one teaspoon) on one hand, and vigorously rub both hands together to warm the oil and your hands.** If you feel any friction between you and your baby during the massage, repeat this step as often as you need.

2. **Hold your hands open with your palms facing your baby.** See Figure 4-1 for an example of how to position your hands.

3. **Make eye contact with your baby and say something like, "Would you like a massage?"**

With your hands open in this way, you are sending your baby your loving energy. Asking her if she wants a massage and creating eye contact engages her and creates a space for bonding. For maximum energy flow, imagine sending love to your baby through the palms of your hands.

Practicing your technique: The Dolphin Stroke

Now that you have all the information you need to get started, we want to give you the opportunity to try out a simple massage technique.

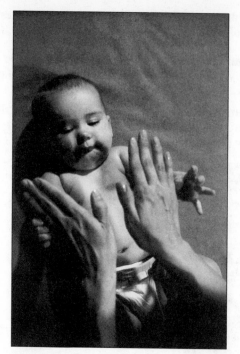

Figure 4-1: Position your hands with your palms facing your baby.

The combination of the oil on your hands and movement in one direction on your baby's soft skin creates a feeling similar to stroking the skin of a dolphin. Hence, the name: The Dolphin Stroke.

This soothing stroke can be used on a baby of any age, including very young babies who need to keep their clothes on during the massage.

Besides being a simple technique for you, this stroke is a gentle way to introduce massage to your baby. It increases the circulation in her body and gives your baby the opportunity to feel and sense all her body parts.

You can use this stroke as a technique by itself, or you may use it to transition between strokes that we detail in Part II of this book. In other words, rather than just moving from one stroke to the next, you can incorporate the Dolphin Stroke in between. Your baby will be very impressed by your finesse as a budding massage therapist.

This stroke can also be used as a finishing stroke — the last stroke used in a series of techniques. Here's how you do it:

1. **Place your left hand (palm down) on the left side of your baby's chest, with your fingers on the front of the shoulder.**

2. **Place your right hand (palm down) on the right side of your baby's chest, with your fingers on the front of the shoulder (see Figure 4-2).**

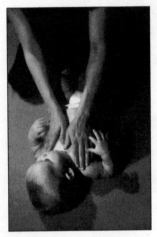

Figure 4-2: Place your hands on each side of your baby's chest, with your fingertips near the shoulders.

3. **Gently glide your hands across your baby's shoulders and down the lengths of the arms, all the way to the hands.**

4. **Repeat steps 1 and 2.**

5. **Glide your hands down through your baby's chest, belly, legs, feet, and toes (see Figure 4-3).**

6. **Repeat this entire sequence three to five times, as your baby will allow.**

If your baby keeps his arms overhead (see Figure 4-4), you can start your stroke from the hands and work down the length of the body, rather than starting at the shoulders and doing the arms separately.

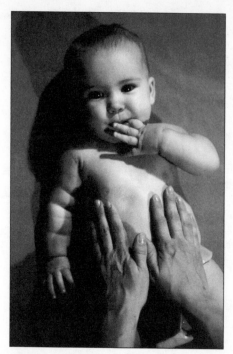

Figure 4-3: Glide your hands down the length of your baby's body.

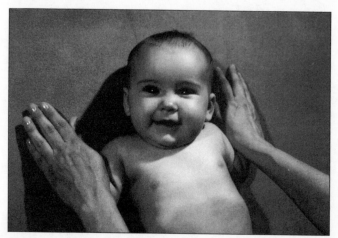

Figure 4-4: Start the stroke at your baby's hands and glide down to the feet.

Part II

Different Strokes for Different Folks: Massaging Baby

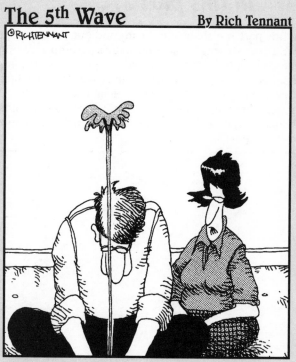

"I would use less pressure when massaging the baby's abdomen."

In this part . . .

In this part, we show you the ins and outs of technique. We cover strokes for all your baby's scrumptious body parts. You get to know what massage terms like *effleurage* and *petrissage* mean, as well as when to use specific techniques on your baby. We give you clear, user-friendly directions for each stroke, and we include lots of photos and illustrations so you can see what we are talking about.

Chapter 5

Massaging the Front Side

. . . .

In This Chapter

▶ Working on the feet and legs

▶ Providing abdominal massage

▶ Using strokes for the chest and shoulders

▶ Massaging arms and hands

. . . .

*W*hile any type of baby massage affords the opportunity to bond, massaging your baby's front side provides a special closeness because you can make eye contact. Your little one will be able to see your face while experiencing your loving touch.

Another benefit of massaging the front side is that very young babies are sometimes uncomfortable lying on their bellies. Because most babies are happy to lay on their backs, you should have no trouble trying out the techniques in this chapter.

As with all the chapters in Part II of this book, we don't expect you to use every technique listed in this chapter every time you massage your baby. (Chances are that he won't stay still long enough for that to happen anyway!) Start by trying one or two techniques — maybe just massage your little one's feet or shoulders. Try the others the next time around. Your baby's interest and stimulation level will determine how many techniques, as well as how many strokes per technique, to use.

And remember that even if your technique isn't perfect, what's most important is for you to stay grounded and present. You achieve this by breathing steadily and keeping eye contact at all times (see Chapter 4). Above all, enjoy what you are doing.

Soothing the Feet and Legs

If this is your baby's first massage, you may want to start with the feet or legs because these areas are less prone to overstimulation than, for example, the belly or chest.

Before you begin a massage, take a look at Chapter 4, which contains essential information about preparing for the experience, asking your baby's permission to massage her, deciding which oils to use, and determining whether your baby is becoming anxious or overstimulated.

When massaging your baby's legs, it's best to perform all the strokes you will be using on one leg before switching to the other leg.

The Taffy Pull

The Taffy Pull is a nice introduction to massage for both of you, as it works only the superficial layer of muscles. This technique is simple and won't overstimulate your baby. In addition, it helps to release relaxation hormones, so don't be surprised if your baby falls asleep. If that happens, you can continue to give the massage if you wish. Just be sure to move slowly and gently, and be ready to offer a warm smile if she wakes up.

The Taffy Pull is an *effleurage stroke,* which means a gentle, gliding stroke. Any effleurage stroke can be used to warm up the superficial muscles, as well as to apply the oil to your baby's body. (After all, you want to apply the oil in a relaxing and soothing way, not just smear it on your baby!) Effluerage calms and soothes the nervous system and is a nice way to begin and end a massage.

Following are the steps involved in The Taffy Pull. Note that you massage just one leg at a time.

1. **Place one hand on the outside of your baby's hip with your palm facing in (see Figure 5-1).**

2. **Move your hand down the outside of her leg to her foot using a gentle gliding stroke.**

3. **When your first hand reaches the baby's ankle, use your other hand to stroke the inside of her leg, starting at the top and moving down.**

4. **Alternate your hands in a continuous motion.** Move your hands continuously to maintain a smooth and rhythmic motion.

If you notice your baby's skin becoming a little red on the surface, this may be an indication that there was some tension in the muscle that was released.

Unless you want a tickle-happy baby, apply a bit of gentle pressure. Find a fleshy part of your own body to practice using different amounts of pressure.

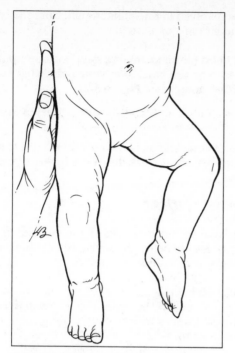

Figure 5-1: Always make sure your palm is facing the baby.

Kneading Dough

This massage works the deeper layers of the muscle. Use this technique after you have warmed up the superficial muscles with a stroke such as The Taffy Pull. Working the deeper layer of muscle removes toxins and increases blood and oxygen circulation, thereby relaxing the muscles. Believe it or not, babies are under a lot of stress: Everything is new to them, and their daily lives are filled with developmental changes. Stress accumulates in your little one's body just like it does in yours. This technique is a gentle way to release some of it.

Kneading Dough is considered a *petrissage stroke,* which is a kneading stroke used on loose, heavy musculature tissue. These strokes often involve lifting, picking, rolling, squeezing, wringing, and kneading. The kneading motion squeezes out toxins in the muscle, moving the waste materials (lactic acid) back into the circulatory system where the waste can be excreted through urination.

Here are the steps involved in Kneading Dough. Note that you massage just one leg at a time.

1. **With one hand (palm facing in), gently scoop up the muscle tissue on the outside of your baby's leg, as if you are kneading dough (see Figure 5-2).**

2. **Continue scooping up the muscle as you work your way down the outside of your baby's leg.**

3. **When step 2 is complete, use your other hand to scoop up the muscle tissue and work down the inside of the leg.**

Squeeze and Twist

The Squeeze and Twist technique works all the muscles in the leg. Because all the muscles are being massaged, this stroke increases circulation and deepens relaxation.

Even though relaxation is the goal, your baby could become stressed by this technique if he becomes too stimulated. If your baby becomes stressed, speak to him in a soothing voice, and stop the massage if you need to.

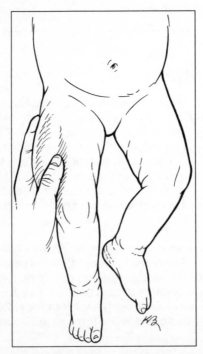

Figure 5-2: Gently scoop up the muscle tissue.

Here are the steps involved in the Squeeze and Twist technique. Note that you massage just one leg at a time.

1. **With both hands, hold onto your baby's leg between your thumbs and forefingers.** One hand is on the outside of the leg (near the hip), and the other is on the inside. Your thumbs are parallel to each other, with little distance between them.

2. **Twist your thumbs and forefingers to your right and then to your left, moving down toward the ankle (see Figure 5-3).** Your hands are moving in opposite directions.

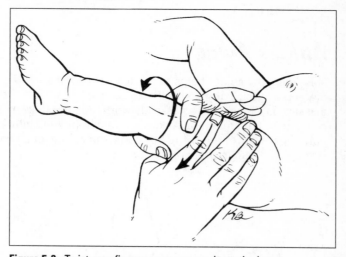

Figure 5-3: Twist your fingers as you move down the leg.

If your baby is enjoying this massage technique, you can also use upward strokes (moving your hands toward the baby's belly). If your baby starts to fuss, simply change the direction of the stroke to move down toward the feet.

Thumb Circles

Like Kneading Dough and Squeeze and Twist, this stroke works the deeper layers of muscle and increases circulation. Using this technique on a very young baby introduces her to a new kind of touch. As with the Squeeze and Twist technique, notice if your baby becomes stressed by the increase in circulation, especially if your baby is very young. If so, stop the massage and use a more soothing technique like The Taffy Pull. Sometimes babies respond unfavorably to being touched in a new way.

Following are the steps involved in using the Thumb Circles technique. Note that you work on just one leg at a time.

1. **Grab onto your baby's thigh with fingers from both of your hands.**

2. **Place your thumbs, side by side, on top of your baby's thigh, near the hip.**

3. **Moving from hip to ankle, make small outward circles with alternating thumbs (see Figure 5-4).**

4. **When you've almost reached the ankle, change direction.** Use alternating thumbs to make outward circles back up the leg.

Ankles Away

Massaging the ankles helps to lubricate the joint and increase the mobility of your baby's foot. If your baby is not walking yet, this massage is a nice way to passively work the joint to keep it lubricated and in full function. Ankles are weight-bearing joints and hold the weight of the entire body. Massaging the joints can strengthen them in preparation for walking.

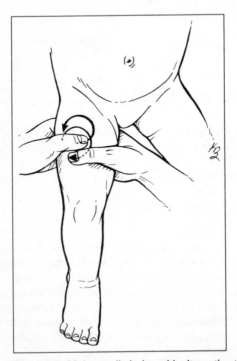

Figure 5-4: Make small circles with alternating thumbs.

Never massage directly on a bone because you can cause your baby pain. Be sure to work around the ankle bone when you do this massage.

Following are the steps involved in the Ankles Away technique. Note that you work on only one ankle at a time.

1. **Cup your baby's ankle in your hands.**

2. **With one forefinger on each side of the ankle, make small circles around the ankle working from the middle of the foot around the ankle bone (see Figure 5-5).**

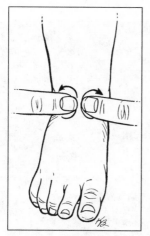

Figure 5-5: Make small circles around the ankle with your forefingers.

This Little Piggy

Each of our feet contains more than 70,000 nerves, which makes them sensitive to stress. You can release stress in your little one's feet by incorporating this stroke into your massage.

Practitioners of reflexology believe that the nerve endings on the bottom of the foot correspond with the organs in the body. Massaging the tip of the pinky toe, for example, can affect one's sinuses. Therefore, a foot massage can become a holistic treatment, improving health throughout the body. Also, in Chinese medicine, all of the *meridians* (energy channels) begin and end on the hands and feet. Therefore, massaging the extremities affects different areas of the body.

Following are the steps involved in doing the This Little Piggy technique. Note that you work on only one foot at a time.

1. **Cup your baby's foot in your hands, and make little circles on top of the foot with alternating thumbs (see Figure 5-6).** For very small babies, use only one thumb.

2. **Continue cupping your baby's foot and stroke down the foot to your baby's toes with your thumbs.**

3. **Grab each toe, one by one, and gently pull (just enough to straighten the toe being pulled).**

4. **Sprinkle your baby's yummy foot with lots of kisses.**

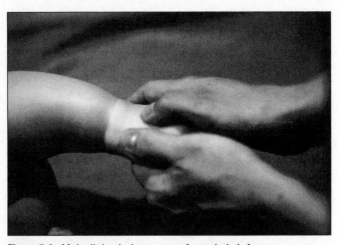

Figure 5-6: Make little circles on top of your baby's foot.

Raking

This stroke is soothing, relaxing, and a great way to end a massage session or get your little one ready for bed.

In baby massage, *finishing strokes* such as this one are used to end the treatment with a sedating effect. These strokes also balance out the entire massage by bringing closure to the treatment. After a while your baby will know that the massage is coming to an end by remembering which stroke you are using.

To perform this technique, use one or both hands, apply gentle pressure, and glide your fingertips down from the top of your baby's leg to the ankle (see Figure 5-7). Note that your hand is simply moving on top of your baby's leg. Use enough pressure so as not to tickle your baby.

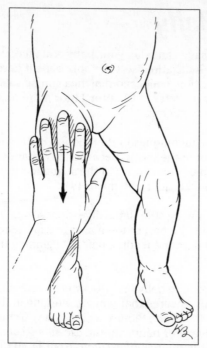

Figure 5-7: Glide your fingertips down the length of your baby's leg.

If your baby becomes a little anxious or cranky, you can use a *touch relaxation* technique: Grab onto both legs and gently shake them to relax the muscles. Be sure to maintain eye contact with your baby and talk with her in a soothing voice.

Combining strokes

Be creative when massaging your baby's feet and legs. When you become comfortable with the techniques we describe here, you won't need to follow our instructions step by step. You'll be able to switch from one stroke to another with ease, and you can combine strokes or even create your own routine to suit your baby.

There is no one right way to massage your baby. Just be aware of whether your strokes are moving toward or away from the heart. Strokes moving away from the heart are less stimulating to your baby.

Relaxing the Belly

Using abdominal massage can relax your baby and increase her digestive functioning. Relaxation isn't the only benefit here; concerns such as constipation, colic, and diarrhea can be safely addressed with massage. Refer to Chapter 11 for more techniques to aid common health concerns.

The goal of each of the techniques in this section is the same: to move stool and gas out of the colon. Because they share common results, you can use these techniques in the sequence shown, switch the order around, or just use one or two.

Massaging your baby's belly stimulates digestion. Assuming you don't want spitting up to be part of the massage experience, we suggest waiting an hour after a feeding before beginning the massage.

Always move strokes on the belly in a clockwise direction. Working in a clockwise direction ensures that you are working in the same direction as the intestinal tract. Picture a clock on your baby's belly. You want to move your hands up the *ascending colon* (from 7:00 to 11:00), across the *transcending colon* (from 11:00 to 1:00), and down the *descending colon* (from 1:00 to 5:00).

Your baby may release gas or have a bowel movement while you are working on this area. These are signs that your massage is working. We suggest that you keep a diaper on or open underneath your baby while working the abdomen, or else have one nearby!

The Water Wheel

The Water Wheel is used to push out any gas or stool that may be stuck in part of your baby's colon. Because your baby's digestive system is still developing, he may have excess gas, especially if he drinks formula. (A breastfed baby can also have trouble with gas if he is allergic or sensitive to certain foods that you eat. The book *Breastfeeding For Dummies* by Sharon Perkins and Carol Vannais [Wiley] contains lots of information about how breast milk and formula can affect a baby's digestive system.) For information on how abdominal massage helps digestion, see Chapter 2.

Following are the steps involved in The Water Wheel:

1. **Place your right hand (pinky side down, palm facing you) just under your baby's left breast, making sure to stay under your baby's ribs.**

2. **Use a paddling motion and stroke down your baby's belly toward the pelvis (see Figure 5-8).**

3. **Switch hands and repeat the first two steps.** Alternate hands, and keep the movements continuous. Be sure to use a little bit of pressure.

Use your baby's reactions as a guide to how much is too much pressure. If she becomes unhappy or looks uncomfortable, make the pressure lighter.

Thumbs to Sides

Thumbs to Sides also pushes gas and stool out of your baby's colon, but this technique works the entire large intestine. This stroke compliments The Water Wheel by addressing the entire colon.

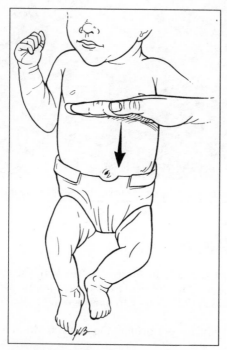

Figure 5-8: Stroke the pinky side of your hand straight down toward your baby's pelvis.

Here are the steps involved in the Thumbs to Sides technique:

1. **Place each hand with the outside of your thumbs down on either side of your baby's belly button. Note that you are only using your thumbs in this stroke.**

2. **Using the outside of your thumbs, stroke out toward your baby's sides (see Figure 5-9).**

Make sure to use a little bit of pressure when using this technique. Watch your baby closely; she will let you know if the pressure is too much.

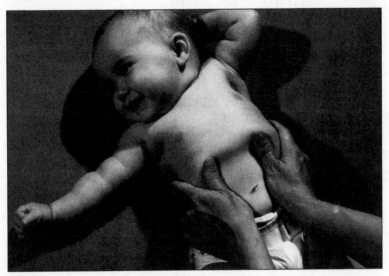

Figure 5-9: Stroke out toward baby's sides using the outside of your thumbs.

Sun and Moon

With this stroke, you are helping Mother Nature with the elimination process. All portions of the colon are addressed in one sweeping movement. This is an efficient way to massage the colon.

Following are the steps for performing the Sun and Moon technique:

1. **Imagine that your baby's belly is a clock.**

2. **Place your right hand at 7:00.**

3. **With your right hand, stroke up and around your baby's abdomen (in a clockwise motion) toward 4:00.** You are making a horseshoe pattern.

4. **Repeat this motion with your left hand (see Figure 5-10).**

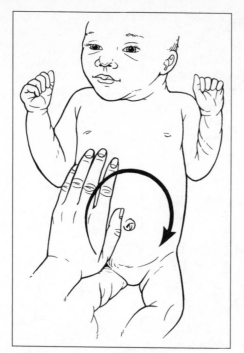

Figure 5-10: Your left hand follows your right hand in a horseshoe pattern.

I Love You

The strokes we've discussed so far in the "Relaxing the Belly" section work the ascending colon first. The I Love You stroke begins working the colon from a different angle. By working the descending colon first, you are releasing pressure that has built in the baby's intestines.

Working the colon from the descending colon first is called *uncorking the bottle*. If you think of the end of the colon as a corked bottle, releasing the cork relieves any pressure that has gathered in the colon.

Here are the steps involved in the I Love You stroke:

1. **Imagine that your baby's belly is a clock.**

2. **Using gentle pressure, start at 1:00 and stroke with one or two fingers straight down your baby's belly to 5:00.** You are making an "I."

3. **Next, start at 11:00 and stroke across to 1:00 and down toward 5:00 with one or two fingers.** You are making an upside down "L" (see Figure 5-11).

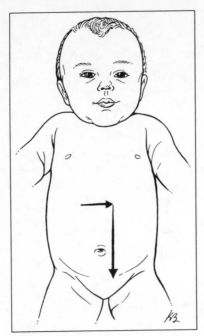

Figure 5-11: With two fingers, make an upside down "L."

> **4. Finally, stroke from 7:00 up, over, and down to 5:00, making an upside down "U."**

Make sure to say "I love you" often as you are doing this stroke.

Opening the Chest and Shoulders

We think it's logical to talk about the chest and shoulders together because the major muscles of the chest attach directly to the shoulders. Bringing the shoulder into a chest stroke creates a nice flow during the massage. Most babies love this.

Massaging the chest increases breathing functions and moves out any congestion that may have accumulated. The shoulder is a ball-and-socket joint, so working the shoulder lubricates the joint and increases range of motion.

Many practitioners of massage and other therapies believe that we hold emotions in our muscle tissues. Even babies can hold feelings and energy around their hearts. Because of this, don't be surprised if you find your baby becoming very stimulated during a chest massage.

The Heart Stroke

The Heart Stroke opens the chest, which makes breathing easier
and relieves congestion from colds. Any stored stress in this area
is pushed back out into the circulatory system and released during
elimination.

Following are the steps you take to perform the Heart Stroke:

1. **Using both hands, make a triangle with your forefingers
   and thumbs by placing your hands palm down on your
   baby's sternum.** Your forefingers are pointed toward your
   baby's chin (see Figure 5-12).

2. **Move the triangle up toward the baby's chin, then separate your hands and move them down around the nipples.**
   You are tracing the shape of a heart on your baby's chest
   (see Figure 5-13).

3. **Finish the shape of the heart by bringing your hands
   together at your baby's belly button.**

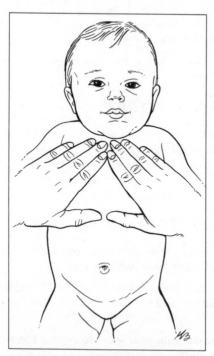

Figure 5-12: Make a triangle with your
forefingers and thumbs.

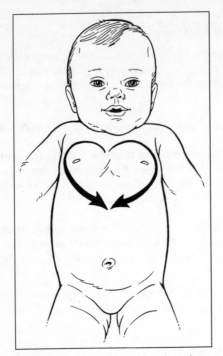

Figure 5-13: Separate your hands and move them down around your baby's nipples.

The Open Book Stroke

The Open Book Stroke stretches and opens the major muscles of the chest and the shoulders. This is a deeper massage because it incorporates joint movement along with stretching. The muscles are elongating, and the shoulder joint is moving within its range of motion.

Here are the steps involved in the Open Book Stroke:

1. **Place both hands palms down on your baby's chest, with your fingers facing your baby's chin.**

2. **Move your hands away from each other, toward your baby's shoulders, and down the length of his arms until you reach his hands (see Figure 5-14).**

3. **Return to the starting position and repeat the stroke as often as your baby will allow.**

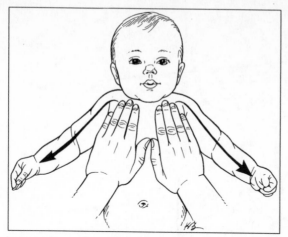

Figure 5-14: Move your hands toward your baby's shoulders and down the length of his arms.

The Butterfly Stroke

The Butterfly Stroke lengthens the major muscles of the chest. The flow of this stroke also includes the top of the shoulders (the *trapezius* muscles), which makes for a smooth and rhythmic stroke.

Following are the steps for performing the Butterfly Stroke:

1. **Place your right hand on your baby's left lower belly.** Your palm should be down and your fingers facing your baby's right shoulder (see Figure 5-15).

2. **Glide your right hand up toward your baby's right shoulder and cup your hand over the shoulder.**

3. **Glide your right hand back to your starting position (the left lower belly).**

4. **As your right hand returns to starting position, your left hand mirrors the stroke.** Start your left hand at your baby's right lower belly and move it toward her left shoulder (see Figure 5-16).

You create a rhythm with this stroke by keeping your hands moving continuously.

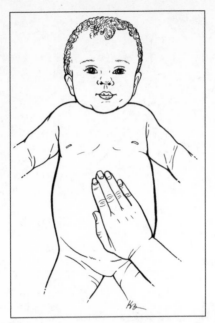

Figure 5-15: Place your right hand on your baby's left lower belly.

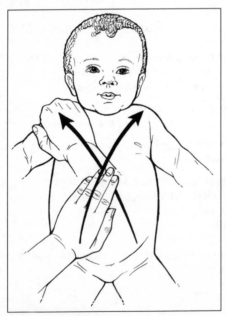

Figure 5-16: Glide your left hand toward your baby's left shoulder.

Reaching for Arms and Hands

Before you know it, your baby starts to use her hands to reach for things, and she begins pulling herself up to practice standing (which means walking isn't far behind). You want to work your baby's hands to help her get ready to use her fine motor skills. Massaging your baby's arms strengthens the muscles so she will be able to pull her body weight up into a standing position. For more information on your baby's development, refer to Chapter 3.

Just as with your baby's legs, we suggest you complete all the strokes you will be using on one arm before switching to the other arm.

Alternating Hands

Alternating Hands is a great stroke to begin working on this part of the body. Like The Taffy Pull (which we describe earlier in the chapter), this is an *effleurage* stroke — it warms the superficial muscles to prepare for deeper work. You want to apply oil to the areas you're massaging.

Here are the steps involved in the Alternating Hands technique:

1. **Place your left hand on the outside of your baby's right shoulder.**

2. **Place your right hand on the inside of your baby's right arm.**

3. **Glide your left hand down toward your baby's hand.**

4. **As your left hand is approaching your baby's hand, your right hand starts gliding down (see Figure 5-17).**

5. **Return to the first step and continue to move your hands in an alternating rhythm.**

The "C" Stroke

This stroke works the deeper layer of the muscles. As you move down your baby's arm, you are wringing any toxins out of his muscles. Because you are twisting in opposite directions and moving across your baby's muscle fibers, you are increasing the relaxation response. For more on stress, see Chapter 2.

1. **With each hand cupped in the shape of a "C," place your fingers around the top of your baby's arm.** Pretend that you are holding tiny cups between your thumb and forefingers.

2. **Gently squeeze and twist your way down your baby's arm to the wrist.** Your hands are moving in opposite directions (see Figure 5-18).

Do not squeeze and twist your baby's wrist.

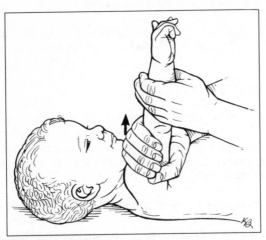

Figure 5-17: When your left hand is approaching your baby's hand, glide your right hand down.

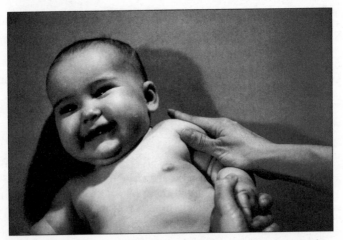

Figure 5-18: Squeeze and twist your hands down your baby's arm in opposite directions.

Wrist work

The wrist is similar to a tunnel, where nerves run through to activate the muscles in the hand. You want to work your baby's wrists to maintain fluidity and free range of movement. Although the wrist is a small area, it contains many nerves, muscles, and bones.

Following are the steps for performing Thumb Circles on your baby's wrists:

1. **Hold your baby's left wrist with both of your hands.** Your baby's palm is facing down.

2. **Using one or both thumbs, make tiny circles on your baby's wrist (see Figure 5-19).**

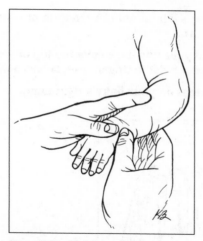

Figure 5-19: Make tiny circles on your baby's wrist with your thumbs.

3. **Turn your baby's hand over, and make tiny circles with your thumbs on the bottom of the wrist.**

4. **Switch hands, and massage your baby's right wrist.**

Hands on hands

Your baby's hands stay clenched until she is ready to use them. Even if your baby's hands aren't in use yet, the act of keeping them clenched creates stress. When your baby does start using her hands to grab objects, the hand muscles are being used constantly, and she is fine-tuning her motor skills. Massaging your baby's hands helps to strengthen, tone, and relax the muscles.

If your baby's hands are clenched, do not try to pry them open. Your baby is still developing and may not be ready to open them. Try to gently stroke or kiss the tops of her fingers to see if they will open.

Hand stroking

This soothing stroke is a good beginning technique, as well as one you can use anytime. Simply holding your baby's hand between yours is comforting and relaxing.

To perform this stroke, use the following steps:

1. **Place your baby's left hand between both of your hands (like a sandwich).**

2. **With the tips of your fingers, stroke the top of your baby's hand from wrist to fingers (see Figure 5-20).**

3. **Repeat these steps on your baby's right hand.**

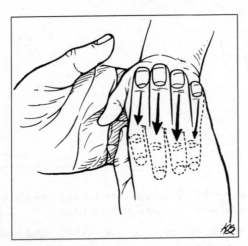

Figure 5-20: Stroke the top of your baby's hand from wrist to fingers.

Finger stroking

There are a lot of joints in the fingers, so it is important to work each finger separately to ensure that each joint is working to its full capacity.

Use these steps for stroking your baby's fingers:

1. **With your thumb and forefinger, grab one of your baby's fingers near the knuckle and gently pull down toward the baby's nail (see Figure 5-21).**

2. **Continue this stroke on each of your baby's fingers.**

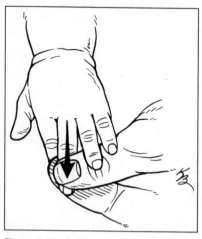

Figure 5-21: Grab your baby's finger with your thumb and forefinger and pull down toward the nail gently.

Chapter 6

Massaging the Face and Neck

In This Chapter

▶ Relaxing muscles around your baby's mouth

▶ Releasing tension around the forehead and eyes

▶ Massaging your baby's ears, chin, and neck

*I*n this chapter, we show you plenty of techniques to relax the muscles in your baby's face. After all, it can be a workout for your little one to feed, laugh, and show off his dimples all day long.

In this chapter, as in Chapters 5 and 7, you should keep in mind that you're free to experiment with the order of the techniques we present. And, of course, you don't have to do them all. You and your baby will figure out together which ones are the most soothing and in what order.

Proceeding with Caution

Before we present all the great techniques you can use to relieve the stress in your baby's facial muscles, we want to offer a few words of caution. Generally, babies are very sensitive about having their heads touched. Because a baby's skull and brain are still developing, the head is a vulnerable and sensitive area. (More than 50 percent of the total growth of your baby's head occurs in the first year of life.) For this reason, we focus in this chapter on the face and neck — areas that most babies enjoy having touched.

In particular, you want to avoid massaging your baby's soft spot — called a *fontanel* — which is where the bones of your baby's skull have not joined completely. The fontanel allows room for your baby's rapidly growing brain to develop. Typically, you can see and feel a pulse in the fontanel. Two spots are usually large enough to be noticeable:

✔ **Posterior fontanel:** Located on the back part of your baby's head. This soft spot should close by 4 months of age.

✔ **Anterior fontanel:** The diamond-shaped soft spot on top of your baby's head, toward the front. Usually, this soft spot closes between 9 and 18 months.

The fontanel is protected by a tough, fibrous membrane, so it is safe to touch and wash the area. But massaging the fontanel is simply too risky.

If you want to include the head in your baby's massage, we recommend light stroking (around — not on top of — the soft spot) only if your baby seems to like the touch. If not, just leave the head out of the massage until your baby begins to enjoy the touch.

Soothing Your Baby's Smile

The muscles in your baby's face hold tension from nursing, sucking, laughing, and teething. Also, each time your baby expresses an emotion, his facial muscles contract to change his expression, which creates tension.

Relaxing the jaw

Your baby's jaw area can contain lots of tension, especially if you have a baby with high sucking needs! The following techniques are easy and useful for relieving stress in the jaw.

Ears to Chin

This is a good beginning stroke to familiarize your baby with the feeling of having your hands on her face. It is a smooth, flowing, and gentle stroke. Use very little pressure; you want your hands to feel like feathers on your baby's skin. If your baby happens to be very sensitive from teething, this stroke may be the only one you can use on her face.

Here are the steps involved in the Ears to Chin technique:

1. **Place your baby on his back, with his feet closest to your body.**

2. **Place your right hand (palm facing baby's head) behind your baby's right ear.**

3. **Place your left hand (palm facing baby's head) behind your baby's left ear (see Figure 6-1).**

4. **Glide both hands (simultaneously) down toward your baby's chin.**

5. **Repeat steps 2 through 4 multiple times, depending on your baby's level of tolerance.**

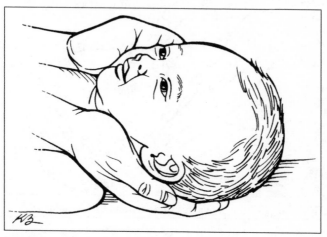

Figure 6-1: Cup your baby's head with your palms.

Small Circles

This massage technique soothes the muscles that babies use for sucking, and it also relieves discomfort from teething. It accomplishes these things by increasing circulation by moving the muscle in all directions, down the length of the jaw line.

Here are the steps involved in the Small Circles technique:

1. **Choose how many fingers to use, depending on the size of your hand compared to the size of your baby's face.** You may use one, two, or three fingers (your pointer, forefinger, and middle finger).

2. **Place one, two, or three of your fingers from your right hand just below your baby's right earlobe.**

3. **Place one, two, or three of your fingers from your left hand just below your baby's left earlobe (see Figure 6-2).**

4. **Make small clockwise circles with your fingers as you move down slowly, following the baby's jaw line.**

5. **You may repeat this sequence three to five times, if your baby likes this technique.**

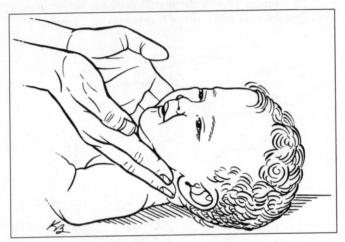

Figure 6-2: Place your fingers just below your baby's earlobes.

Tapping the Jaw Line

Tapping along the jaw line helps to sedate the sensitive nerve endings in your babies gums and to increase circulation in this area. This technique can soothe your baby's discomfort from teething, sucking, and crying. Here are the steps to take:

1. **Place the forefinger and middle finger of your left hand under your baby's left earlobe (palm side in).**

2. **Place the forefinger and middle finger of your right hand under your baby's right earlobe (palm side in) — see Figure 6-3.**

3. **Swiftly tap your fingers (from both hands) alternately down your baby's jaw line.** In other words, one finger from each hand is touching your baby's jaw line at a time. Be sure to use gentle pressure.

4. **When you reach the bottom of the jaw line, tap your fingers back up your baby's jaw to the earlobes.**

5. **Repeat this sequence three to five times.**

A variation of this stroke is to tap both fingers from each hand at the same time, down and back up your baby's jaw line.

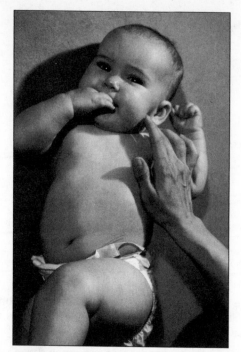

Figure 6-3: Place your fingers just below your baby's earlobes.

Loving those sweet cheeks: The Smile Stroke

Your baby uses a lot of facial muscles to express emotions such as wonder, pleasure, frustration, and anger. You can use massage to relax and soften the muscles of the face.

You're probably aware that it takes more muscles to frown than to smile. If your baby pouts or frowns frequently, this is a great stroke to use to relax your baby's upper lip and cheeks. Here's how:

1. **Place your left thumb (palm facing in) just under your baby's left nostril.**

2. **Place your right thumb (palm facing in) just under your baby's right nostril.**

3. **Using both thumbs, stroke outward toward the apples of your baby's cheeks (see Figure 6-4).**

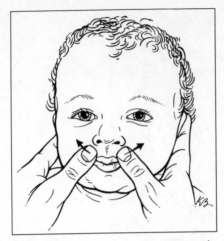

Figure 6-4: Stroke your thumbs out toward your baby's cheeks.

4. **Continue to glide your thumbs up toward your baby's temples.** Imagine you are drawing a happy face on your baby (see Figure 6-5).

5. **If your baby allows, repeat this sequence three to five times.**

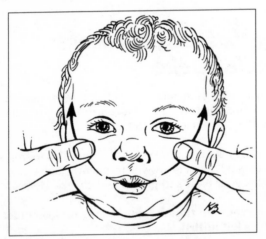

Figure 6-5: Draw a smile on your baby's face.

You can complete the smile by repeating the sequence but beginning with your thumbs just under your baby's lower lip.

Relaxing the Eyes

When you think of muscles, the eyes may not leap to mind. But we all use our eye muscles to express emotion, which can create tension.

If your baby tends to move around a lot, make sure that you move very slowly when you attempt this massage technique, and proceed with great caution.

Following are the steps for the Circling the Eyes technique:

1. **Place the forefinger of your left hand on the left side of the bridge of your baby's nose.**

2. **Place the forefinger of your right hand on the right side of the bridge of your baby's nose.**

3. **Simultaneously, gently sweep your forefingers down the bridge of your baby's nose (see Figure 6-6).**

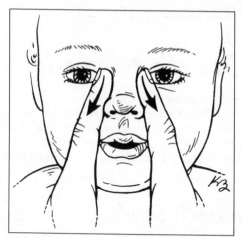

Figure 6-6: Sweep your fingers down the bridge of your baby's nose.

4. **Move your fingers down and out underneath the lower eyelids.**

5. **Glide your forefingers up and around the top of your baby's eyebrows (see Figure 6-7).**

6. **Your fingers will meet in between baby's eyebrows.**

7. **Repeat this sequence three to five times, if your baby allows.**

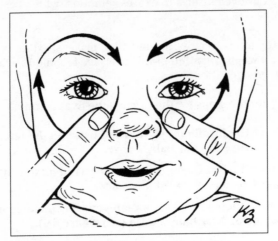

Figure 6-7: Glide your fingers up and around.

Smoothing Out the Forehead

Your baby's forehead can be very expressive, showing emotions like surprise or wonder, or indicating a serious state of mind. Consequently, your baby's forehead can also hold a lot of tension in times of distress, especially if you have a colicky baby. It's a good idea to make massaging your baby's forehead a part of your routine.

The Open Book Stroke

This stroke smoothes and relaxes the muscles of the forehead. There are two variations.

Following are the steps for the first variation of the Open Book Stroke:

1. **Place the fingertips (palms down) of both your hands in the center of your baby's forehead (see Figure 6-8).** The tips of your fingers are just below your baby's hairline.

2. **Simultaneously glide your hands slowly away from one another, out to the sides, across your baby's forehead (see Figure 6-9).**

3. **Repeat this sequence three to five times if your baby likes it.**

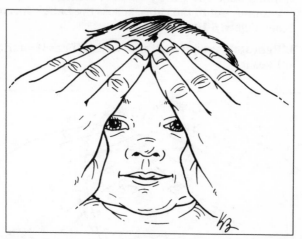

Figure 6-8: Place your fingertips just below your baby's hairline.

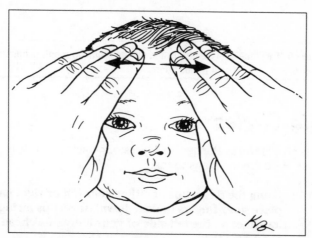

Figure 6-9: Glide your hands across your baby's forehead.

Here are the steps for the second variation of this stroke:

1. **Place the fingertips (palms down) of both your hands in the center of your baby's forehead, midway between the hairline and eyebrows.**

2. **Simultaneously glide your hands slowly away from one another, out to the sides, across the baby's forehead — see Figure 6-10.**

3. **Repeat this sequence three to five times if your baby likes it.**

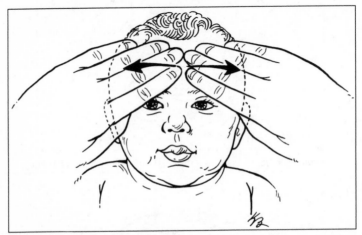

Figure 6-10: Place your fingertips midway between your baby's hairline and eyebrows and glide your hands apart.

Big Circles

This stroke works the deeper layers of muscles that lie in the forehead. Here are the steps to take:

1. **Using the fingertips of either your left or right hand, place your fingers (palms down, fingertips facing the hairline) on the left side of your baby's forehead (see Figure 6-11).**

2. **Move your fingers in a clockwise circular motion, moving from the hairline down toward the eyebrows (see Figure 6-12).**

3. **Repeat steps 1 and 2 three to five times if you can.**

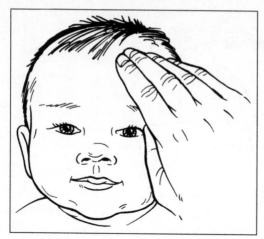

Figure 6-11: Place your fingertips on the left side of your baby's forehead.

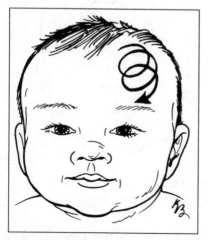

Figure 6-12: Move your fingers in a circular motion toward the eyebrows.

4. **Using either the fingertips of your left or right hand, place your fingers (palms down, fingertips facing the hairline) in the center of your baby's forehead.**

5. **Move your fingers in a clockwise circular motion, moving from the hairline down toward the eyebrows (see Figure 6-13).**

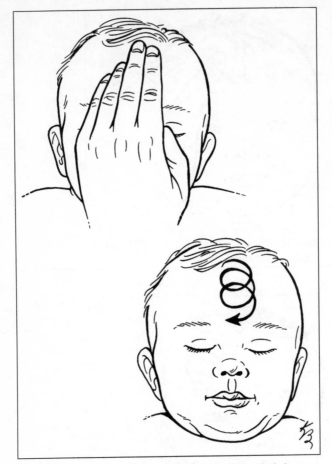

Figure 6-13: Place your fingers in the center of your baby's forehead and circle your fingers down toward the eyebrows.

6. Repeat steps 4 and 5 three to five times if you can.

7. Using the fingertips of either your left or right hand, place your fingers (palms down, fingertips facing the hairline) on the right side of your baby's forehead.

8. Move your fingers in a circular motion, moving from the hairline down toward the eyebrows (see Figure 6-14).

9. Repeat steps 7 and 8 three to five times if you can.

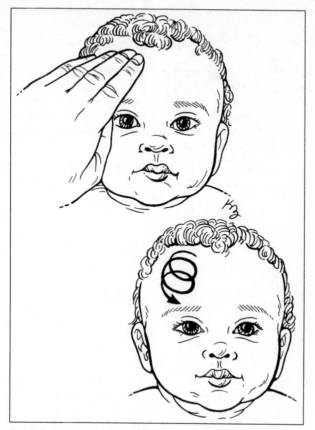

Figure 6-14: Place your fingers on the right side of your baby's forehead and circle your fingers down toward the eyebrows.

The Temple Stroke

The muscles located on the side of your baby's forehead hold a lot of tension, which can create headaches. The Temple Stroke can help your baby relax and relieve any tension in this area.

Here are the steps involved in the Temple Stroke:

1. **Place your right fingertips (palm side in) on your baby's right temple.**

2. **Place your left fingertips (palm side in) on your baby's left temple.**

Ear infections

Many babies and children are plagued with ear infections. Ear infections typically affect the middle ear and the *Eustachian tube* — a long tube that connects the ear to the nose and throat, allowing fluids to drain out of the middle ear. Babies are particularly susceptible to infections because the Eustachian is short and horizontal. If fluids build up in the middle ear (usually from a sinus or respiratory infection), bacteria can grow and create an infection.

It can be difficult to identify what is wrong with a preverbal baby, but here are some common symptoms of an ear infection to look for:

- Fussiness

- Crying

- A slight fever

- Pulling or tugging at the ear lobes

- An unwillingness to suck on a pacifier or bottle, or to nurse

- A recent bout with a cold or sinus infection

- Diarrhea

- An unpleasant odor coming from the ear

Most ear infections aren't serious, and they do go away as your baby grows older. However, babies with chronic ear infections are at risk for ear drum damage or hearing loss.

Antibiotics are sometimes used to treat ear Infections. New guidelines for treating ear infections suggest using a pain reliever first and administering antibiotics only if the infection doesn't improve. If your baby isn't in too much pain, you can help to improve the infection with massage. Try a gentle massage along the back of the ear, down along the jaw bone, and in front of the ear using a circular motion with one or two fingers. You can also use a gentle massage on the back of your baby's head, near the base of the skull. These techniques can help clear the fluid out of the Eustachian tubes to improve healing.

If you want to treat the infection with alternative therapies, acupuncture and chiropractic care have been successful in treating and preventing ear infections. Also, if you breastfeed your baby for at least six months, your baby's chances of getting ear infections are lessened due to the immune-building antibodies that are present in breast milk.

3. **Move the fingertips of both hands in a circular, clockwise motion (see Figure 6-15).**

4. **Create six small circles.**

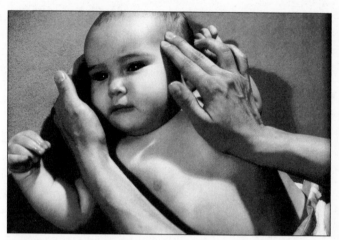

Figure 6-15: Move your fingertips in a circular, clockwise motion.

While you're using this technique, make your movements smooth and flowing to increase your baby's relaxation. (The same holds true for all the techniques in this chapter.)

Paying the Ears, Chin, and Neck Some Attention

At first glance they may seem incidental, but the ears, chin, and neck hold tension and energy too! Don't forget to devote some time to each during your massage.

The Ear Stroke

Following is a simple technique to use on your baby's ears:

1. **With your left thumb and forefinger, gently take hold of your baby's left earlobe.**

2. **Roll your baby's earlobe between your fingers, using a kneading motion (see Figure 6-16).**

3. **Do this technique for three to five seconds.**

4. **With your right thumb and forefinger, gently take hold of your baby's right earlobe.**

5. **Repeat steps 2 and 3.**

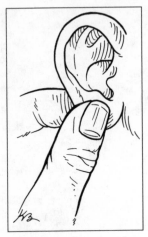

Figure 6-16: Use a kneading motion to roll your baby's earlobe between your fingers.

Chinny Chin Chin

Your baby's chin is an extension of the jaw line, which means there are a lot of muscles in this area that contain tension because of nursing, crying, and laughing. Here are the steps involved in this stroke:

1. **Place the pads of the fingers from your left hand on the right side of your baby's chin.**

2. **Place the pads of the fingers from your right hand on the left side of your baby's chin (see Figure 6-17).**

3. **Create small circles with your fingers.** The fingers of your left hand move in a counterclockwise direction, and the fingers of your right hand move in a clockwise direction. Move your hands away from each other (see Figure 6-18) and up along the jaw line.

4. **Move your fingers back down the jaw line to your starting position.**

5. **Repeat the sequence three to five times in each direction.**

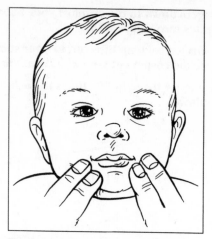

Figure 6-17: Place your fingers on both sides of your baby's chin.

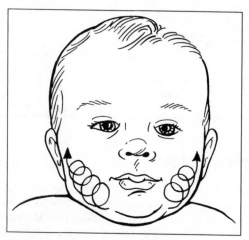

Figure 6-18: Move your hands away from one another as you create small circles.

Here's a variation of the Chinny Chin Chin stroke:

1. **Place the pads of the fingers from your left hand on the right side of your baby's mouth.**

2. **Place the pads of the fingers from your right hand on the left side of your baby's mouth.**

3. **Move your fingers down to the point of your baby's chin with small circles (see Figure 6-19).**

4. **Continue the circles back up the chin to your starting position — near the corners of your baby's mouth.**

5. **Repeat this sequence three to five times in each direction, if your baby allows.**

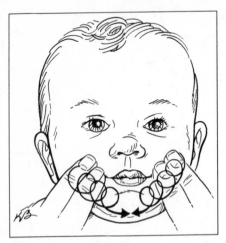

Figure 6-19: Starting with your hands on either side of your baby's mouth, circle your fingers down your baby's chin.

Working the neck

Think of what an enormous burden it must be for your baby to support his big, heavy head! As your baby develops more neck strength, tension and stress can be held here too. Massaging your baby's neck releases tension and makes it easier for him to learn new movements.

The strokes we describe here can be used anytime, even when your baby is sitting or lying on your lap. On very young babies, it is difficult to even find their neck, so you can skip these techniques until your baby is about 6 months old.

Small Circles

This stroke massages your baby's lymph nodes. Here are the steps to follow:

1. **Use your left hand and place the pads of your fingers just below your baby's right ear.**

2. **Make small circles with your fingers in a clockwise direction.**

3. **Move your fingers down your baby's neck, all the way to the collar bone (see Figure 6-20).**

4. **Repeat steps 1 through 3 with your right hand, beginning under your baby's left ear.**

5. **Repeat the entire sequence three to five times if possible.**

With this technique, you can work one side of the neck at a time or both sides simultaneously. A nice variation is to start the circles at the back of your baby's ears and work down toward the back of the neck.

Scooping

The following technique creates length and space in the muscles of the back of your baby's neck. Done correctly, it feels great. However, be certain to *gently* grab onto your baby's neck!

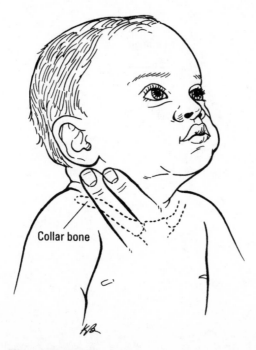

Collar bone

Figure 6-20: Move your fingers in a clockwise direction, down toward the collar bone.

1. With either your right or left hand, gently pinch the back of your baby's neck between your thumb and forefinger and lift up the skin and muscle.

2. Repeat this motion three to five times if your baby allows.

Chapter 7

Massaging the Back Side

- -

In This Chapter

▶ Massaging the backs of the legs

▶ Using different positions

▶ Relaxing your baby's bottom

▶ Soothing the neck and shoulders

- -

*B*efore you know it, your baby is rolling over, laying on her belly, and trying to crawl. In this chapter, we invite you to take advantage of your baby's natural curiosity and growing abilities to move her body.

In addition to showing you how to massage the back of your baby's body, we supply tips to make your massage experience the best it can be and suggest ways to incorporate massage into your daily activities.

Taking Advantage of Tummy Time

Unless you have been practicing yoga regularly for many years, your baby is much more flexible than you! He can bend his back forward, backward, and sideways, and he can twist around to see what's going on behind him.

Besides providing agility, the many muscles of your baby's back help to protect his spine and keep his body upright. Using massage to ease the tension and stress out of your baby's back and neck muscles will not only make him more comfortable but will help him maintain good posture as he develops and matures.

If your baby has been trying to stand or walk , you can imagine how much stress his body experiences with each attempt (and tumble!). Massage is a good way to make the exciting adventure of standing and walking smoother for your baby.

TIP

Many babies under 6 months are uncomfortable lying on their bellies for very long. You can use different positions to massage your baby's back, such as having him sit in your lap or holding him on your shoulder. You don't have to postpone massaging your baby's back until he begins to enjoy tummy time!

Massaging the Legs and Feet

It's good to massage the back of your baby's legs because of the connection between the lower back and the *hamstrings* — the muscles in the back of her legs. If the hamstrings become tight, your baby may experience some discomfort in the lower back.

As your baby begins to practice standing, she is using muscles that haven't been used before. Massaging the muscles on the back of the body increases your baby's body awareness.

The techniques that you can use to massage the back of the legs and feet are essentially the same techniques we discuss in Chapter 5 for massaging the front of the legs and feet. Here, we show you how to use these techniques on the back of the body.

The difference is your baby's position while you massage her. Whereas the only option for massaging her front side is to have her lie on her back, here you have a few options:

✔ Place your baby sideways (belly down) on your lap (see Figure 7-1). This position is wonderful because you can literally massage your baby anywhere!

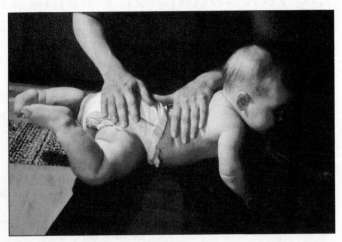

Figure 7-1: Lay your baby on her belly sideways on your lap.

✔ Place your baby on his belly on a flat surface, such as a bed, changing table, or soft carpet (see Figure 7-2).

✔ Lean your back against a wall or piece of heavy furniture for support. Place your baby belly down between your legs, with her head near your feet (see Figure 7-3).

This is a great position to use if you've had a cesarean section or have any other health condition that makes it difficult for you to stand.

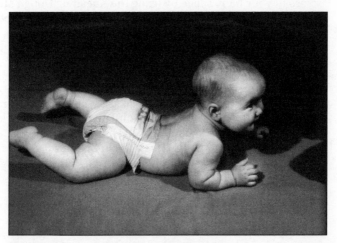

Figure 7-2: Lay your baby down on a flat surface.

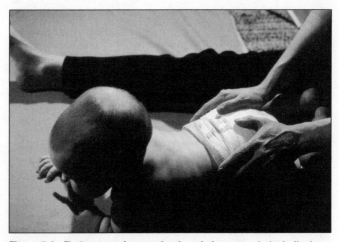

Figure 7-3: Find support for your back and place your baby belly down between your legs.

The Taffy Pull

Use this gliding stroke to warm up the muscles (see Figure 7-4). Refer to Chapter 5 for the steps involved.

Kneading Dough

As we explain in Chapter 5, you can gently release accumulated stress in your baby's legs by using the Kneading Dough stroke. Figure 7-5 shows how to perform this stroke on the back of the legs.

Thumb Circles

The Thumb Circles stroke is great for increasing circulation in your baby's legs. However, when you massage the back of your baby's legs, be sure not to use deep pressure on the back of the knee because of the veins and nerves that are in this area. Figure 7-6 shows how this technique, described in Chapter 5, can be used on the back of the legs.

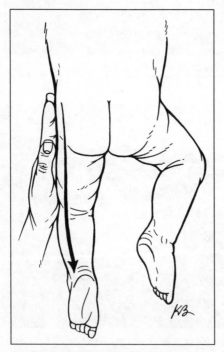

Figure 7-4: Glide your hand down from your baby's hip to the ankle.

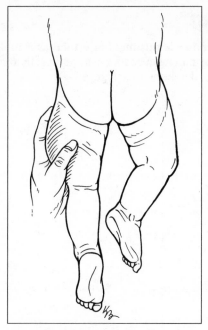

Figure 7-5: Gently scoop up the muscle
tissue as you work down the leg.

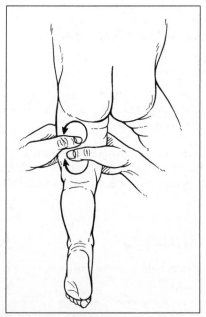

Figure 7-6: Make small outward circles
with alternating thumbs.

Ankles Away

As we describe in Chapter 5, this technique increases mobility in your baby's feet. Remember never to massage directly over a bone; massage around the ankle bone (see Figure 7-7).

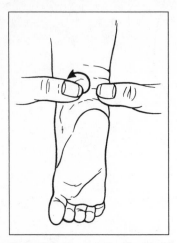

Figure 7-7: Use your forefingers to make small circles around the ankle bone.

Bottoms Up! Kneading Your Baby's Bottom

The largest muscles in anyone's body are the *gluteus maximi* — the muscles commonly known as the buttocks. (See, no one is picking on you — everyone's got a big backside!)

The buttocks are the muscles that propel your baby when he walks, and they are the muscles that connect the back and legs together. Your baby uses these muscles a lot: when he sits, lays, walks, and even crawls.

Alternating Thumbs

You can release the tension held in your baby's bottom with this simple stroke.

1. **Place your thumbs side-by-side on the top of one of your baby's cheeks (near the lower back).**

2. **Moving from the top of the buttock down toward the crease of the leg, make small outward circles with alternating thumbs (see Figure 7-8).**

3. **Repeat the first two steps on your baby's other cheek.**

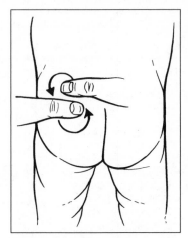

Figure 7-8: Make small outward circles with alternating thumbs.

Circular Palmer

This is a great stroke to use if you have a baby who is mobile. By bracing your hand against her hip, you are helping to keep her still until she learns to relax into the massage.

1. **Hold your left hand palm side in, and brace your baby's left hip.**

2. **Place your right hand palm down on your baby's right cheek with your fingers facing your baby's head.**

3. **Use your whole palm to make small counterclockwise circles down your baby's buttock (see Figure 7-9).**

4. **Hold your right hand palm side in and brace your baby's right hip.**

5. **Place your left palm down on your baby's left cheek with your fingers facing your baby's head.**

6. **Use your whole palm to make small counterclockwise circles down your baby's buttock.**

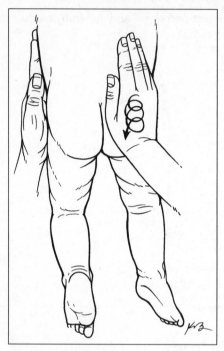

Figure 7-9: Make small circles using your whole palm.

Keep one hand on your baby at all times. Doing so ensures that your baby feels you, even though she can't see you!

The Large Bottom Stroke

The name of this technique describes the stroke used — it isn't for large bottoms only!

1. **Place your right hand on your baby's right cheek with your palm down and fingers facing your baby's head.**

2. **Place your left hand on your baby's left cheek with your palm down and fingers facing your baby's head.**

3. **Stroke your baby's bottom using the entire palm of both hands if possible.** Alternate your hands by moving your right hand in a clockwise direction and your left in a counterclockwise direction (see Figure 7-10).

4. **Repeat this stroke as often as your baby likes.**

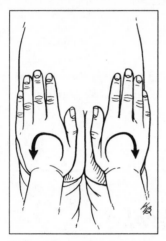

Figure 7-10: Make large circles with your palms.

Finger stroking

This is a relaxing technique to use as a finishing stroke during your massage. Here are the steps involved:

1. **Place your right hand on the top of your baby's right cheek, with your palm down and fingers facing your baby's head.**

2. **Place your left hand on the top of your baby's left cheek, with your palm down and fingers facing your baby's head.**

3. **Gently stroke down each cheek with both of your hands (see Figure 7-11).**

4. **Immediately repeat steps 1 through 3 to maintain a smooth flow.**

5. **Repeat this sequence as often as your baby likes.**

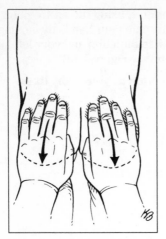

Figure 7-11: Stroke your fingertips down each of your baby's cheeks.

Doing the Back Stroke

Have you noticed how perfect your baby's posture is? Slouching is learned behavior; babies naturally sit up straight and tall when their muscles are strong enough to support sitting. Regular massage helps to maintain your baby's perfect posture — plus, you can give your baby a back massage anywhere!

When we talk about the anatomy of the spine, we typically divide it into three segments: the *cervical spine* (where most movement occurs), the *thoracic spine,* and the *lumbar spine.* Below the lumbar spine lies the *sacrum,* which is part of the pelvis.

Each segment of the spine is made up of vertebrae that are separated by discs, which act as cushions. There are seven vertebrae in the cervical spine, twelve in the thoracic spine, and five in the lumbar spine (see Figure 7-12).

The spine develops from birth through young adulthood — it usually completes its development around 18 years of age. You never want to massage directly on your baby's developing spine. The techniques we describe in this section all involve massaging around the spine.

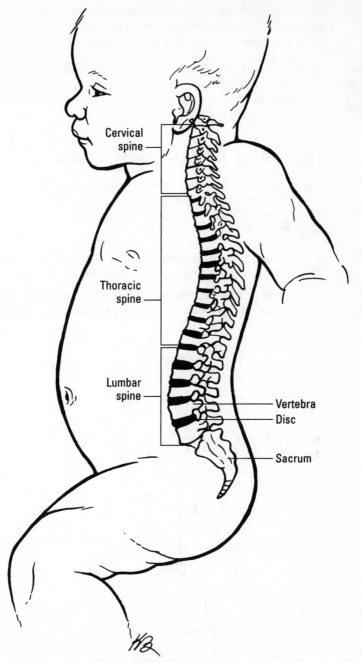

Cervical spine

Thoracic spine

Lumbar spine

Vertebra

Disc

Sacrum

Figure 7-12: The anatomy of the spine.

The next time your little one gets bored in the waiting room of the doctor's office, place her sideways on your lap and massage her back. You'll see how fast that fussy behavior goes away!

Depending on the direction of your movements, a back massage may be stimulating or sedating. Try moving your hands toward the buttocks to quiet your baby, or move the strokes toward your baby's head for a stimulating massage.

The Long Effleurage Stroke

This stroke is a fact-finder, meaning it gives you the opportunity to become familiar with the muscles in your baby's back and where she may be holding tension. You may also use this stroke to apply oil to your baby's back.

1. **Place both your hands palm side down on your baby's back, with your fingertips near the shoulders.**

2. **Stroke both hands gently down the back toward the sacrum, just above your baby's buttocks (see Figure 7-13).**

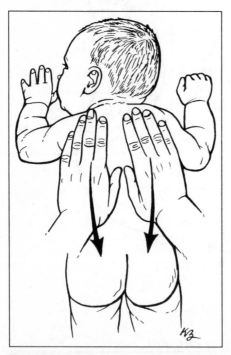

Figure 7-13: Stroke both hands down your baby's back.

3. **Stroke both hands gently back up the back toward your baby's neck.**

4. **Repeat this sequence three to five times.**

For maximum relaxation, glide your palms smoothly over your baby's back in one sweeping motion.

Back and Forth

With this stroke, you are working against the grain of the muscle fibers, which really helps to warm up the muscles, as well as to reduce tension.

1. **Place both hands palms down perpendicular on your baby's back, near the neck (see Figure 7-14).**

2. **Alternate moving your palms in a sawing movement down your baby's back (see Figure 7-15).**

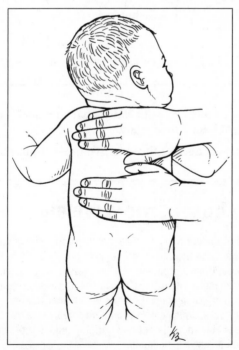

Figure 7-14: Place both hands perpendicular on your baby's back.

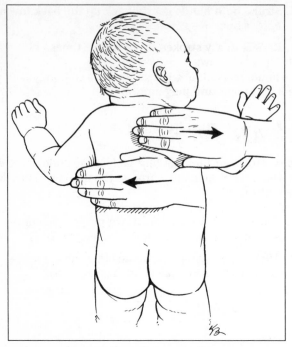

Figure 7-15: Move your palms in a sawing movement down your baby's back.

3. **Work your hands up your baby's back toward the neck, and repeat back down again.**

4. **Repeat this sequence three to five times if possible.**

Using front carriers wisely

If you are considering wearing your baby, we suggest that you use a sling (which we discuss in Chapter 1) because the sling protects your baby's spine by keeping his weight evenly distributed. We like front carriers (such as Baby Bjorns) too, but prolonged use (a few hours or more a day) may place too much stress on your baby's spine and create a condition called *spondylolisthesis,* which occurs when one vertebra slips over another vertebra, causing a lot of pain. To safely use a front carrier, make sure that your baby is able to hold her head upright, and keep the length of time your baby is in a front carrier to a minimum.

Swooping

You can use this easy stroke anywhere to soothe, relax, and quiet your baby. Here's how:

1. **Place one hand perpendicular on your baby's back, near the neck.**

2. **Place your other hand, palm down, over your baby's buttocks.**

3. **Swoop your hand down your baby's body, from the neck to the butt, as if you are petting a dog or cat (see Figure 7-16).**

4. **You can vary this technique by placing one hand on your baby's ankles instead of the buttocks, and swoop down from the neck to the ankles (see Figure 7-17).**

5. **Repeat this sequence three to five times if possible.**

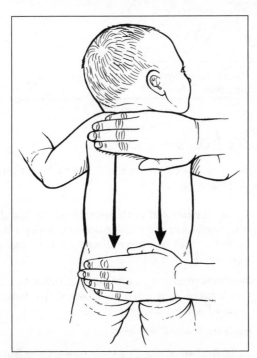

Figure 7-16: Swoop your hand down toward your baby's buttocks.

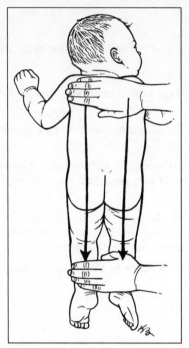

Figure 7-17: Swoop your hand down from the neck to the ankles.

Small Circles

This stroke helps you work some of the deeper layers of the back muscles. Here are the steps to take:

1. **Place the finger pads of both your hands facing down, with your hands perpendicular on your baby's back. Your fingertips will be above the spine, beginning at the neck area (see Figure 7-18).**

2. **Using medium pressure, make small clockwise circles with your fingers, and work your way down toward the buttock (see Figure 7-19).**

3. **Work back up toward the neck.**

4. **Repeat the first step, but this time place your fingertips underneath your baby's spine.**

5. **Repeat steps 2 and 3.**

6. **Repeat this sequence three to five times.**

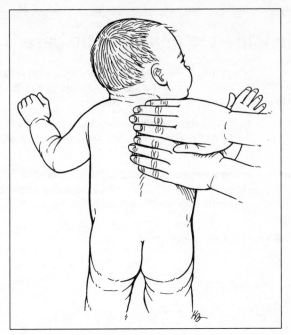

Figure 7-18: Place your fingertips above your baby's spine, near the neck.

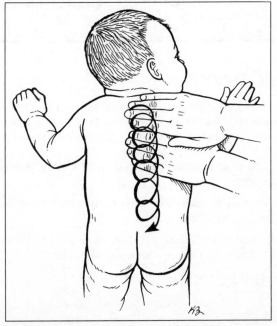

Figure 7-19: Make small clockwise circles with your fingertips.

INFANT WISDOM

Considering chiropractic care

Chiropractors adjust *subluxations* in the spine, which are partial dislocations in the spinal vertebrae. When the vertebrae dislocate, the nervous system is affected, which can affect tissues and organs throughout the body.

Subluxations can occur in babies and children as a result of a difficult birth, tumbles and falls during the crawling and walking years, falls from learning to ride a bicycle, and emotional stress.

Adjusting or manipulating the spine places the misplaced vertebrae back into place. Gentle chiropractic adjustments are safe for babies' fragile and developing spines and have been effective in aiding common discomforts in babies and children, such as the following:

✔ Earaches and frequent ear infections

✔ Bed wetting

✔ Colic

✔ Frequent crying

✔ Constipation

✔ Allergies

✔ Breathing difficulties

To locate a pediatric chiropractor in your area, go to the International Chiropractic Pediatric Association's Web site at www.icpa4kids.com.

Sacral stroke

The *sacrum* is a triangular-shaped bone located just below the lumbar spine and just above the buttocks. This is a great stroke to use to alleviate constipation. Plus, it feels nice to your baby!

1. **Place your thumbs, palm side down, on either side of the sacrum.**

2. **Alternate thumb circles over and around the sacrum (see Figure 7-20).**

3. **For a nice variation, you can make the circles in either a clockwise or counterclockwise direction.**

4. **Repeat the sequence three to five times.**

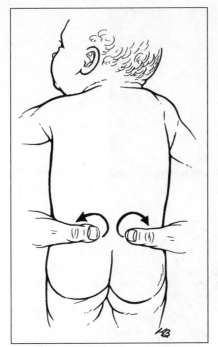

Figure 7-20: Circle your thumbs over and around the sacrum.

Raking

This is a nice finishing stroke, as it tends to produce a sedating effect if the sequence is repeated a couple of times.

1. **Place one hand, palm down, near your baby's neck with your fingers facing toward your baby's head (see Figure 7-21).**

2. **Comb or gently rake your fingers down toward the buttocks.** Keep in mind that you don't want to massage directly over the spine.

3. **Add a variation by starting at your baby's head and raking down toward the feet.**

4. **Make the pressure of the stroke lighter as you continue.**

5. **Repeat the sequence as often as you both like (or until one or both of you fall asleep!).**

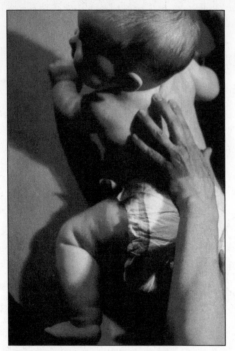

Figure 7-21: Place one hand on your baby's back.

Relaxing the Neck and Shoulders: Long Strokes

In Chapter 6 we show you how to massage your baby's neck. Here we show you how to massage both the neck and shoulders in one technique.

This stroke creates space between your baby's ears and shoulders by elongating the muscles in the neck. You can use this stroke even though your baby's neck is not very long!

If you have a lap baby, take advantage of your baby's natural curiosity to look around by incorporating this stroke whenever her head is turned to one side.

1. **Place the finger pads of your right hand just below your baby's right ear.**

2. **Place the finger pads of your left hand just below your baby's left ear.**

You can choose to work both sides of the neck simultaneously or one at a time.

3. **Using one long soothing movement, gently stroke down the sides of your baby's neck, all the way to the shoulder area (see Figure 7-22).**

4. **Repeat this sequence as often as you and your baby like.**

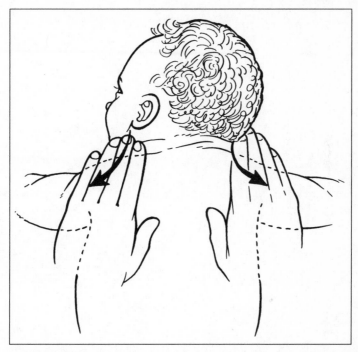

Figure 7-22: Use one long flowing stroke down the sides of your baby's neck.

Part III

Making Massage Part of Your Baby's Life

The 5th Wave   By Rich Tennant

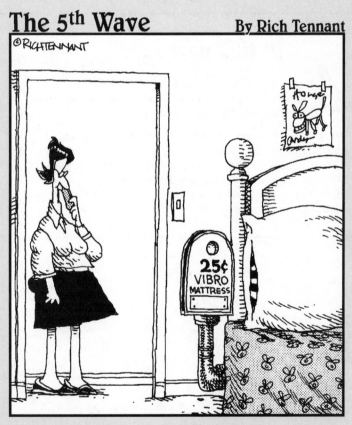

"He doesn't like to sit still for massages any more, so I came up with an alternative."

In this part . . .

All babies and families are different. In this part, we explain how and when to take the techniques from Part II and apply them to your baby.

We provide detailed information on how to massage a preemie, newborn, or toddler — including one who would rather be mobile than sit still, even for your loving touch! And we suggest many ways to bring massage into your daily life — on the changing table, in the bathtub, around nap time, and more.

Chapter 8

Preemies and Newborns

. . . .

In This Chapter

▶ Touching your baby in the hospital

▶ Handling your preemie with care

▶ Massaging your newborn

▶ Making sure that your baby is thriving

. . . .

*I*n this chapter we show you how you can incorporate touch and massage into your routine and relationship with your baby even before you leave the hospital. We pay close attention to special considerations for premature babies, and we discuss how to make sure your baby is thriving.

Handling an Early Arrival

A healthy full-term pregnancy lasts approximately 40 weeks. Babies born anywhere between 38 and 42 weeks are usually developmentally normal. Babies born prior to 36 weeks are considered premature and may have physical problems, such as the following, that require longer hospital care:

✔ An inability to breathe properly

✔ Difficulty retaining heat and staying warm

✔ An inability to breastfeed

✔ Underdeveloped lungs

Despite these potential complications, babies born after 32 weeks typically have a high survival rate with few long-term effects.

Keep in mind that babies born prematurely look different than babies born at term. Their skin can be very red, and you may be able to see the blood vessels through their skin because their bodies haven't yet developed fat.

Risks for premature labor

Sometimes babies just come early, and there isn't anything that you could have done differently to prevent it. However, following is a list of some risk factors that can increase the possibility of having a premature labor. If any of these risk factors apply to you, talk with your doctor about how to address them so you can reduce the risk of a premature birth.

✔ Giving birth to multiple babies (such as twins or triplets)

✔ Smoking during pregnancy

✔ Being malnourished during your pregnancy

✔ Having a health issue such as diabetes or high blood pressure

✔ Experiencing high levels of stress during pregnancy

✔ Using drugs or alcohol during pregnancy

✔ Dealing with a health concern during pregnancy such as *placenta previa* (where the placenta covers part of the cervix) or *preeclampsia* (whose symptoms include high blood pressure and protein in the urine).

✔ Having a previous premature baby

✔ Being underweight or overweight during your pregnancy

✔ Having an infection with a fever during your pregnancy

When a baby is born prematurely, the experience can be very stressful — possibly even traumatic — for both you and your baby. Here are some of the reasons why:

✔ Your baby is not developmentally or emotionally ready for life outside of the womb.

✔ Your baby may have serious health concerns.

✔ Your labor was undoubtedly stressful and may have been delayed with the use of medicine that slows down uterine contractions.

✔ You may not feel emotionally ready to be a parent.

✔ You may not have had a chance to physically prepare for your baby's arrival by setting up the nursery or installing the car seat.

In addition, when a baby is born prematurely, you don't experience the normal process of welcoming your newborn into the world.

Premature babies need special care, which begins as soon as the delivery is complete. For example:

✔ Instead of being handed to you right away, your baby may be taken for tests immediately.

✔ You may have to be moved to a different hospital in order to be placed in a neonatal intensive care unit (NICU).

✔ Bonding between you and your baby may be interrupted due to an early separation in the hospital. Premature babies are often placed in incubators, where they are kept warm and given the opportunity to further their development.

✔ You may even have to leave the hospital without your baby.

 The hospital where your coauthor Ilene works is one of the few medical centers that offers a nurturing touch program in its NICU. This means that a trained and qualified provider teaches caretakers and parents how to be involved and to bond with a premature baby. If your baby comes early, we recommend that you ask your healthcare provider if a similar program is available in your area.

Finding time for touch in the hospital

If you and your baby have been moved to the NICU, the hospital staff will explain how and why you need to touch your baby. If you are reading this section to prepare for the possibility of a preterm baby, or if you don't need to be transferred to the NICU, we show you what you need to know.

Benefiting your preemie

Your premature baby experiences plenty of benefits from receiving your touch, including the following:

✔ Increases in weight gain

✔ Improved breathing patterns

✔ Stabilized heart rate

✔ Stabilized body temperature

✔ Decreases in stress levels

✔ Improved sensory awareness

✔ Improved sleep patterns

✔ Less chance of developing touch aversion, which some premature babies develop due to their sensitivity to touch and uncomfortable experiences in the hospital

Premature babies are often isolated upon birth, unlike other babies, which is why incorporating touch right away is so important! Research conducted by the Touch Research Institute (see Chapter 1) indicates that, on average, premature babies who are massaged gain almost 50 percent more weight and are released from the hospital at least six days earlier than premature babies who are not massaged.

Benefiting the caregiver (that's you!)

Your baby is not the only one who benefits from your touch. When you have a premature baby, you get the following benefits from touch as well:

✔ You have an opportunity to bond with your baby.

✔ You have support from the hospital staff and the team that is working with your special family.

✔ Your baby is able to come home with you sooner!

✔ You feel more confident and able to take care of your premature baby.

Bonding with your preemie

Even though your baby may be separated from you, it is still possible (and important!) to create a warm and loving environment for your preemie that facilitates bonding. Here are some suggestions:

✔ If your baby is in an incubator, take some receiving blankets and sleep with them for a night. The next day, roll them up and place them around your preemie so she begins to associate your smell with feeling safe and held.

✔ Talk to your baby often! Your preemie has heard your voice for months and will feel reassured by hearing it now. You can softly sing lullabies, too.

✔ Pump and store your breast milk. (For guidelines on storing breast milk, see www.lalecheleague.org.) If you are separated from your baby, pumping will keep your breast milk supply flowing.

Because your baby was born early, your breast milk will be different than if your pregnancy went full term — it will contain different nutrients and be a different consistency. However, your milk will still help your baby's developing immune system.

Using three types of touch

When you have a premature baby, the hospital staff shows you three basic types of touch you can use. Your doctors will recommend which type of touch is best for your baby, depending on your baby's size, age, and medical status.

At this stage, any nurturing touch is beneficial to both you and your baby. By including touch in your baby's first days and weeks, you are creating a foundation for a stronger, healthier baby who will thrive from massage!

Here are the three basic types of touch you will use:

✔ **Hand containment:** Simply lay your hands on your baby while he is in the incubator. Depending on the position of your baby and your baby's ability to tolerate touch, you may be able to hold his head in the palm of one hand while your other hand rests on your baby's bottom or belly. Or you may introduce touch just by placing one hand (or a couple of fingers) on your baby.

A firm touch is more beneficial (and easier tolerated!) than a light ticklish touch.

This is typically your baby's first introduction to touch. By experiencing hand containment, your baby begins to find your touch and smell familiar and feels more safe and secure each time you touch him.

Containment helps your baby hold his energy. Preemies and newborns need help containing their energy because they lack any control over their bodies. It seems like there isn't a relationship between body parts in very young babies; they are loose and limp. Young babies also haven't yet learned skills to deal with stress and emotions. Any time your baby is in a position similar to being in the womb, he is "held together," and his energy is contained.

Babies who are able to contain their energy are more able to be organized, meaning they are able to regulate their systems and stay balanced. Organized babies are more focused, learn faster and easier, and cry less often. This is because their energy is used for developing, learning, and growing.

✔ **Kangaroo care:** When you've been given the okay to remove your baby from the incubator (usually for short periods of time in the beginning), you may place her on your bare chest. (You probably want to have her in a diaper!) The name *kangaroo care* comes from the way a kangaroo mother feeds her baby.

Having close contact with the caregiver regulates a premature baby's breathing and heart rate. In this position, your baby also is affected by your body warmth, which increases your attachment.

Kangaroo care helps mothers and fathers feel more bonded and capable as parents. Also, mothers who use kangaroo care with their premature babies tend to be more successful with breastfeeding.

✔ **Nurturing touch:** As your baby grows, you will be able to incorporate more touch into his experiences. While you are in the hospital, your touch will be mostly about holding your baby and having skin-to-skin contact. This type of touch is important to create a foundation of safe and nurturing contact for your baby that will later build into a massage.

Moving slowly

Premature babies come into the world before their neurological systems have fully developed. The reason babies are first held instead of touched is for containment (which we explain in the previous section). Because their neurological systems aren't fully developed, premature babies may not be able to handle touch. Containing their bodies and energy gives them the safe, secure feeling they experienced in the womb.

Don't be discouraged if your baby reacts negatively to your touch. Just remember to move slowly and be patient. Your patience will pay off as you watch your baby become more active, alert, and responsive to your touch.

Continuing contact when you get home

When your baby is well enough to go home with you, it is important to continue the skin-to-skin contact and holding techniques.

Move softly and slowly. Just a few minutes (or even seconds) of some kind of tactile stimulation and nurturing touch, such as holding, rocking, or massaging, will do you and your baby a world of good!

Creating a positive experience

Here are some tips to make massage and nurturing touch for your preemie a good experience for both of you:

✔ Keep your movements slow and gentle.

✔ Don't use any oils yet. You may use warm water to reduce the friction of your hands on your baby.

✔ Keep your baby very warm. You may want to massage your baby with his clothes on (see the upcoming section "Providing contact through clothing").

✔ Start the massage on your baby's legs, or on her fingers and toes. These areas of the body are less stimulating and are non-invasive. You may even begin just by holding these areas of the body.

✔ Avoid upward strokes (those that move toward the head). They may be too stimulating to your preemie. Keep your strokes moving in a downward (toward the feet) direction.

✔ Your baby will probably be very stimulated by a back massage, so avoid this area until your preemie is able to tolerate the stimulation of a massage on the front of the body.

✔ Try to avoid too light of a touch. Tickling your baby is very stimulating!

✔ As your baby becomes stronger, you can begin to massage her buttocks while you are holding her. Just lightly rubbing your full palm over her whole butt will suffice.

✔ Most of your touch with your baby will be given while he is lying on your chest in a reclining position. Your baby will most likely be too small to lie by himself on a bed or on the floor.

✔ Keep the lights and your voice low. Avoid using music until your preemie is less easily stimulated.

✔ Maintain eye contact and reassure your baby with positive affirmations like, "Mommy (or Daddy) is here, and everything is okay."

Your preemie may be so tiny that you can only touch him with a finger. That's okay: Use your judgment and follow his cues (which we discuss next) to give him the level of stimulation he needs.

Responding to your baby's cues

While you are in the hospital, you have two key ways of knowing if your baby becomes overstimulated. First, you can observe that she has a negative response; see Chapter 4 for a discussion of the cues that indicate a baby is overstimulated. Second, the monitors she's hooked to keep track of your baby's vital signs.

Failure to thrive syndrome

When you bring your baby to your pediatrician for well-baby visits, your doctor documents your baby's weight, length, and head circumference and compares his development with other babies his age using a growth chart. If a baby is not growing or loses weight, he may be diagnosed with *failure to thrive syndrome.* Your physician will track when the lack of development occurs and help you find ways to encourage your baby's growth.

With a premature baby, a *corrected age* may be used to plot his growth. The corrected age is figured by subtracting the number of weeks of prematurity from the postnatal age. Growth charts are available just for premature babies, but they may not be reliable due to the small number of premature babies used to compile the statistics. Whichever method your doctor chooses (to adjust the baby's age or to use a preemie growth chart), make sure she uses it consistently.

Most premature babies catch up to the growth of other newborns by the age of 2.

When you come home from the hospital, you no longer have the benefit of monitors, so you must keep a close eye on your baby's reactions to touch. By now you should have a good idea of how much stimulation is too much and how your baby responds if she is overstimulated.

If you see that your baby is becoming overstimulated, change her environment by reducing the amount of stimuli:

- ✔ Dim the lights.

- ✔ Stop talking or singing.

- ✔ Quiet other noises in the room, such as the television, the radio, and people talking or coming in and out of the room.

- ✔ Hold your baby without moving your hand(s) across her body.

Welcoming Your Newborn Bundle of Joy

Preemies aren't the only babies to benefit from skin-to-skin contact and touch. Here are some suggestions to help you provide touch for your newborn in the hospital:

✔ Ask the delivery room nurse to place your newborn on top of your bare chest as soon as possible after delivery so you can immediately have skin-to-skin contact.

After natural childbirth, a newborn placed on your chest will most likely crawl to your nipple and begin to suck.

✔ Ask your healthcare provider to delay tests and vaccinations for as long as possible (approximately one hour) so you can have more immediate bonding time with your baby. (See the sidebar "Routine hospital tests" for a rundown of the procedures that take place shortly after delivery.)

Holding your baby just after birth increases the production of *oxytocin* and *endorphins,* the hormones that create mothering feelings and increase attachment.

✔ Use this early bonding time to gaze into your baby's eyes. You'll be surprised at how alert he is!

The more time you spend with your newborn in the hospital, the stronger your attachment will be, and the greater your sensitivity toward your baby's needs and cues will be.

Routine hospital tests

Just after birth (and hopefully after a little mother–baby bonding time), the hospital performs routine exams, tests, and vaccinations on your baby. Here are some of the most common procedures:

✔ The Apgar test: Designed to determine whether your baby needs to be closely monitored, the Apgar measures heart rate, breathing, color, muscle tone, and response to stimulation.

✔ Vitamin K shot: Because newborns may be deficient in vitamin K, it is routine to give babies an injection that aids in blood clotting and reduces the risk of abnormal bleeding.

✔ Eye ointment: An antibiotic is put into your baby's eyes to prevent any germs that she may have had contact with during labor from causing an infection.

✔ Blood tests: Most hospitals test for your baby's blood type, Rh factor, sickle cell disease, phenylketonuria (PKU), hypothyroidism, and galactosemia. Many hospitals routinely check for other diseases as well.

✔ Hearing screening test: Many hospitals routinely offer hearing screening tests immediately after delivery.

Rooming in

You'll have an easier time incorporating touch and strengthening your attachment with your baby in the hospital if you elect to *room in* — meaning that your baby stays in the hospital room with you rather than in the nursery. You may be unsure about making this choice because you will need to rest after labor. However, while you are in the hospital, the staff does routine visits around the clock for your entire stay, so you really won't get the rest you need until you get home. Keeping your baby in the room with you makes it easier for you to touch, hold, cuddle, and feed him as much as your little one needs.

Providing contact through clothing

If you deliver a healthy, full-term baby, you can actually begin to use simple massage techniques while you're in the hospital. However, keep in mind that newborns, like preemies, are sensitive to over-stimulation. For this reason, it's a good idea to keep your baby's clothes on when you first begin to massage.

Why can removing a baby's clothes cause overstimulation? There are several possible reasons:

- ✔ Very young babies lose heat rapidly. They simply feel too cold and uncomfortable with their clothes off.
- ✔ Removing clothes from a very young baby can be difficult. Because your baby doesn't have control of his head, slipping a onesie off an infant or preemie is hard!
- ✔ Many babies seem to feel vulnerable with their clothes off.

If you massage your baby with his clothes on, you also don't have to worry about using oils or finding the right place to do your massage.

A good stroke to start off with in the hospital is the Dolphin Stroke (see Chapter 4), which is easy to do and relaxing for your baby.

Establishing a massage routine at home

The easiest way to make massage part of your newborn's life is to establish a routine early. It's easy to do: Simply set aside a few minutes in your day for massage. If you can create a regular time to give your baby a massage, she will begin to look forward to it —

even to expect it! In Chapter 10, we show you how to incorporate massage into daily or weekly rituals, such as changing diapers and bathing.

When you first bring your newborn home, we suggest that you use the techniques we describe in Chapter 5, beginning with your baby's legs. These techniques are easy to use, less stimulating than some of the others in this book, and noninvasive. You can use any of them on your baby while keeping her clothes on.

Your coauthor Joanne has been massaging her baby, Ava, since birth. As I write this, Ava (at 7 months) "asks" for a massage by going into position: lying on her back with her arms up over her head and making eye contact. She nearly always does this after a bath (our regular massage time) and on the changing table.

Because she has been receiving regular massages since she was born, Ava is able to tolerate a full massage (to both the front and back sides of her body) without becoming overstimulated. In fact, the massage relaxes and grounds her. (See the sidebar on "Grounding.")

Using touch while you nurse your baby

In the early weeks of your baby's life, much of his awake time will be spent eating. If you are breastfeeding, be prepared to nurse your baby every two to three hours around the clock. If you are using formula, feedings occur less frequently (because formula isn't as easily digested as breast milk) — around every three to four hours.

INFANT WISDOM

Grounding

To be *grounded* means to be fully present in the moment. Your energy is down low in your body. You are aware of your feelings, your thoughts, and the people around you, and you feel your feet on the ground.

You can tell that your baby is grounded when she seems settled, alert, and focused.

To ground yourself, take a look at the section on "Keeping your own stress level in check" in Chapter 2. While you practice the breathing technique described there, remove your shoes and stand with your legs hip width apart. Bend your knees a little and tip your pelvis forward slightly. As you breathe, visualize your energy moving down through your body and through your feet. Imagine that you are connected to the earth through your feet.

The advantages of breastfeeding

Breastfeeding offer many benefits to both you and your baby. We certainly recognize that everybody's situation is different, and for some women (due to health issues, work schedules, or other concerns), breastfeeding is out of the question. But if breastfeeding is possible for you, or if you are on the fence about whether to breastfeed or use formula, keep these things in mind:

 ✔ Breastfeeding significantly reduces the risk of you developing breast cancer.

 ✔ Breast milk is more easily digested than formula and produces less allergies in your baby.

 ✔ Breast milk contains antibodies that boost your baby's immune system.

 ✔ Breast milk is free!

 ✔ Your uterus will shrink back to its normal size faster if you breastfeed.

 ✔ Breastfeeding burns approximately 500 to 1,000 calories a day.

 ✔ Breast milk helps premature babies "catch up" faster!

 ✔ Breastfeeding releases hormones that help mothers relax.

For much more information about breastfeeding, see *Breastfeeding For Dummies* by Sharon Perkins and Carol Vannais (Wiley.)

Nursing is quiet time that you spend cuddling, loving, and feeding your baby all at once. You can nurse your baby whether you are breastfeeding or using a bottle. Dads can nurse their babies, too!

If you are breastfeeding, and/or if this is your first baby, you may need some time to settle in and become used to feeding your baby. After the two of you become familiar with nursing and it becomes second nature, you can incorporate touch into your nursing schedule.

During your baby's first weeks and months, you are building up to giving him a full massage.

Here are some tips for incorporating nurturing touch while you nurse your baby:

 ✔ While holding your baby, use a free hand to stroke down your baby's body.

 ✔ If you are breastfeeding in a side-lying position, you can make small circles on the bottom of one of your baby's feet using your thumb. When you switch to the other breast, massage the bottom of your baby's other foot.

✔ If she can tolerate having her head touched, lightly stroke your baby's head and gaze into her eyes as she nurses.

✔ If you are bottle-feeding your baby (with breast milk or formula), your partner can become part of the bonding experience by stroking your baby's legs, feet, and hands while she eats.

It's not a bad idea if your partner massages *you* during nursing as well. New parents need rest and relaxation, too!

If you are just too exhausted from late night feedings and new parenthood in general to even think about massage while you're feeding the baby, take care of yourself and just rest during nursing. There will be plenty of time for massage as your baby develops.

Adding to Your Massage Routine

Throughout this chapter, we provide suggestions for incorporating massage into your preemie's or newborn's life without overstimulating him. At this point, you may be asking, "How do I know when I can increase the amount of massage time and add more techniques to the routine I'm already using?"

Here are some pointers to answer that question:

✔ When your baby's muscles and facial expressions are relaxed during the massage, that means he's comfortable with what you're doing and may be ready for more.

✔ With your preemie or newborn, introduce only one or two new techniques at a time. This way, you are better able to gauge her stimulation level before it's too late and she's overstimulated. Plus, you'll be able to keep track of which specific techniques are overstimulating.

✔ If you have used only downward strokes on your baby so far, try one of the techniques that uses an upward stroke, and watch your baby's reaction.

✔ If you have tried most (or all) of the techniques for the front side of the body (see Chapter 5) and your baby doesn't become overstimulated, *and* if your baby likes to lay on his tummy, you may want to try out techniques on the back side of the body (see Chapter 7).

✔ When your baby begins to enjoy having his head and face touched, introduce some of the techniques we show in Chapter 6.

Chapter 9

Older Babies and Toddlers

In This Chapter

▶ Keeping your child's interest

▶ Creating rhymes and introducing games

▶ Making massage a family affair

▶ Using massage to set limits with your toddler

*I*n earlier chapters, we caution you to be sure to keep your baby's stimulation level to a minimum if possible. In this chapter, we change our tune. With older babies and toddlers, you need to use stimulation to keep their interest so they'll stay still long enough to receive a massage.

In this chapter, we include some information about your child's development — particularly about her growing interest in play and games — to help you be creative in finding ways to stimulate your baby or toddler during the massage. We suggest incorporating rhymes and games into massage time, as well as bringing other family members into the mix. Finally, we discuss how you can use massage to help set limits with your toddler.

Holding Still: Keeping Your Child's Interest

Do you remember the days when you knew where your baby was every second (because you were holding her almost all the time)? Now your baby is constantly on the move, and your time and energy is spent making sure that your house is child-friendly and your little one doesn't get bored. Sometimes you may long for the good old days, filled with lots of quiet cuddle time!

If you have been massaging your baby since infancy, you'll have an easier time now getting her attention and holding it long enough for a massage. For babies who are experienced at receiving massages, it is just part of the daily routine, much like taking a bath. However, now that she is older, you need to be creative and introduce some fun ideas to keep her interest.

If you bought this book so that you can begin massaging your 2-year-old, your task of keeping her still long enough for a massage will be challenging, but the rewards will be great. Be patient, and know that whatever touch you bring to her at this age will benefit both of you.

Massaging your older baby

When we refer to an *older baby,* we're talking about a child who is 6 to 12 months old. In this section, we show you some behaviors you can expect to see in your older baby and ways to incorporate his interests during a massage.

Anticipating your baby's development

Here are some developmental milestones and interests you can expect to see from your older baby:

- ✔ Your baby spends less time on your lap and becomes more interested in his environment.
- ✔ He starts to crawl probably between the ages of 6 and 9 months, and shortly thereafter he begins pulling himself up to stand.
- ✔ He becomes more interested in his body and loves to put his toes in his mouth.
- ✔ Your baby grabs everything within reach!
- ✔ He notices when you leave and is becoming shy around strangers.
- ✔ His language is developing, so you hear a lot of cooing and babbling.
- ✔ Your baby begins teething.

Occupying your baby during a massage

To continue to fit massage into your baby's day, our best advice is to get creative. You know your baby best; use whatever she is interested in to keep her attention. Here are some examples:

- ✔ Babies love encouragement as they learn to do new things. While your baby is learning to crawl, give her a few minutes to practice while you encourage her. When she becomes frustrated, reward her attempts and ease her frustration with a massage.

✔ Older babies love to see their reflections in mirrors. You can place your baby (who can now sit on her own!) in front of a floor-to-ceiling mirror and massage her neck and shoulders or back while she laughs at her reflection.

✔ Teething may cause serious discomfort for your baby at this stage. You can massage your baby's gums (see Chapter 11) and cheeks (see Chapter 5) to ease the teething pain.

✔ Older babies love to put things in their mouths. Give your baby a safe teething toy while she is on her back, and let her suck away while you massage the front side of her body.

Incorporating rhymes into massage

Most older babies love rhymes. They are just beginning to practice their language skills, and they love to play games with words. Rhymes can help keep your baby interested as you give a massage, and an added bonus is that you are teaching your baby language and rhythm at the same time.

Following are two examples of rhymes that you can sing or chant during the massage. They each refer to movements that you can incorporate into the massage.

You can choose from literally hundreds of children's rhymes. If you're in the mood to learn some new ones, we suggest a quick search on the Web. For example, you can find lyrics to many children's songs and nursery rhymes online at www.mamalisa.com.

Roll Over

There were three on the bed

And (your baby's name) said,

"Roll over, roll over."

(Roll your baby over and begin massaging the other side.)

So they all rolled over and one fell out.

(Roll your baby over again, or keep him on that side for the massage.)

There were two on the bed

And (your baby's name) said,

"Roll over, roll over."

So they all rolled over and one fell out.

(Roll your baby over again, or keep him on that side for the massage.)

There was one on the bed

And no one said,

"Roll over, roll over."

Horsey Horsey

Horsey, horsey don't you stop

Just let your feet go clippety clop.

The tail goes swish

(Roll your baby onto her belly and massage her bottom.)

And the wheels go round.

Giddy up, we're homeward bound.

Ain't in a hurry, ain't in a scurry,

(Slowly roll your baby onto her back and massage the front side.)

We'll be on our way. Hey!

Horsey, Horsey on our way,

We'll be traveling many a day.

The tail goes swish

(Roll your baby onto her belly and massage her bottom.)

And the wheels go round.

Giddy up, we're homeward bound.

(Pull your baby up to sitting or standing, and finish with a hug.)

Massaging your toddler

A toddler is 12 months to 2 years old. In this section, we show you some behaviors you can expect to see in your toddler and ways to incorporate her interests during a massage.

Toddlers have a natural curiosity and a short span of attention. Limit your massages to just a few minutes, and you will find it easier to keep your toddler's attention.

Anticipating your toddler's development

Here's what you can expect to see during this age:

- ✔ Your baby has transformed into a walking (and falling!) toddler.
- ✔ She is your little helper — eager to try to dress herself and do things around the house.

- *No* is her favorite word.
- She parrots everything you say.
- Your older toddler can run and climb.
- She loves physical games.
- Your older toddler loves to jump and practice gymnastics.
- She enjoys creating art and playing with shapes.

Incorporating rhymes and songs into massage

As with an older baby, you can use rhymes and songs to try to keep your toddler's interest during a massage. Your toddler will want to be part of the action whenever possible, so consider saying or singing rhymes that encourage him to interact. For example, you may want to try "If You're Happy and You Know It."

If You're Happy and You Know It

If you're happy and you know it, clap your hands. *(clap clap)*

If you're happy and you know it, clap your hands. *(clap clap)*

If you're happy and you know it, then your face will surely show it.

If you're happy and you know it clap your hands. *(clap, clap)*

You can incorporate the body parts you wish to massage by changing the verse to something like, "If you're happy and you know it touch your leg."

If you don't feel like hearing your own voice all the time, you can also sing along with your toddler to popular children's music while giving him a massage. CDs such as these are fun to sing along to:

- *Peter, Paul, & Mommy* by Peter, Paul, and Mary (Warner Brothers)
- *Free to Be. . .You and Me* by Marlo Thomas and Friends (Arista)
- *All You Need Is Love: Beatles Songs for Kids* by Various Artists (Music for Little People)
- *Singable Songs for the Very Young: Great with a Peanut-Butter Sandwich* by Raffi (Rounder Records)
- *Beauty and the Beast: Original Motion Picture Soundtrack* by Various Artists (Disney)

Reading books during massage

If you are not yet reading to your toddler on a regular basis, we strongly recommend it! You can use reading time to give your toddler a massage. Place your toddler in your lap and let her turn the pages for you while you give her a massage.

If you need some suggestions for classic kids' books to have in your library, here are just a few:

- *Are You My Mother?* by P.D. Eastman
- Any stories by Dr. Seuss
- *Where the Wild Things Are* by Maurice Sendak
- *Goodnight Moon* by Margaret Wise Brown
- *Will You Be My Friend? A Bunny and Bird Story* by Nancy Tafuri

Unless your toddler has been receiving massages regularly for a while, she may be stimulated by the massage and not ready to go to sleep immediately afterwards. Avoid massaging your toddler before bedtime if this is the case.

Playing games during massage

With a little creativity, you can make massage a game. Here are some ideas to get you started:

- Play "Simon says" and tell your toddler to stay still while mommy massages his shoulders.
- Play horsey by letting your toddler bounce on your knee and massage his back while he bounces away.
- Play hide-and-seek with the rule that whoever gets caught receives a massage.
- Ask your toddler to lie on his belly over a beach ball, and give him a back massage. Encourage him to have fun bouncing and rolling on the ball before and after the massage.

Another way you can sneak a massage into your toddler's day is to catch him while he is watching his favorite video.

Making Massage a Family Affair

So far in this book, we've focused on massage as a one-on-one experience between a parent or caregiver and a child. But you can use the massage techniques and ideas we suggest in this book to encourage stronger bonds between siblings and the entire family. In this section, we explain how to accomplish this goal.

Including your older child

If you have older children, we encourage you to include them in the giving and receiving of massages. Here are some benefits:

- ✔ You can keep a sibling's natural jealously toward a new baby to a minimum.

- ✔ You teach your children how to give and receive nurturing and compassionate touch.

- ✔ The bond between the siblings is enhanced.

- ✔ You may be able to take a much-needed break!

 The bond between siblings is a strong one, and massage can help make it stronger. Although many siblings have ups and downs in their relationship from childhood to adulthood, the bond typically outlives the parental relationship and lasts longer than most marriages.

If you're going to ask your older child to give your younger one a massage, obviously you need to keep in mind the age and abilities of the older child, along with your younger child's needs. For example, you may be able to teach a 7- or 8-year-old some of the more complicated techniques we cover in this book (like The Taffy Pull we describe in Chapter 5), but younger children need to stay with easier techniques (like the Dolphin Stroke we show in Chapter 4).

Here are some tips for getting an older sibling started with massage:

- ✔ Have your older child choose which massage technique he loves the best and let him be "in charge" of giving your younger child that particular massage.

- ✔ Have your child practice his technique on you first, so you can help him determine the right amount of pressure to use.

- ✔ Encourage your child to practice massage strokes on her favorite doll.

 If the sibling giving the massage is fairly young, we strongly recommend that you supervise the massage at all times. Children may not be able to read cues of overstimulation (which we discuss in Chapter 4), and they may use too much pressure during the massage. Both children involved in the massage may need you to guide them and make sure that the touch they are giving and receiving is safe and loving.

Getting creative with family massages

If you want to include more members of your family in the giving and receiving of massages, that's terrific. There really isn't one particular way to make that happen because everybody's family is different. We encourage you to experiment and find the best way for everyone in your family to benefit.

Here are some ideas that may help get your creative juices flowing:

- ✔ While one parent is reading a toddler or older baby to sleep, the other can give her a massage.

- ✔ During TV time, have siblings take turns giving each other massages, and the parents can do the same.

- ✔ Use massage to give a step-sibling the opportunity to bond and connect with a new baby.

- ✔ Encourage massage during family vacations. A new schedule — even a fun one — can throw everyone's sleep patterns off, so use massage as a way to bring relaxation and quiet time into your vacation plans.

Using Massage to Your Toddler's Advantage

Toddlers struggle to reconcile their need for autonomy with their need for their parents' help and guidance. One of the many ways that kids in this age group express their autonomy is by saying *no*. Sometimes toddlers say *no* to everything, even things that you know they want. You may find that your toddler says he doesn't want a bowl of cereal, for example, only to turn around and demand that same bowl a few seconds later.

Your job as a parent or caregiver is to set limits and boundaries for your toddler. You may sometimes doubt this, but it's good for your toddler to experience the frustration of not getting everything he wants and to have limits set. At the same time, it's good for you to respect your toddler's *no*. Listening and responding to your toddler's words teaches him that he has power in the world and some control over his environment.

How to protect your child from sexual abuse

Because the incidence of childhood sexual abuse is so prevalent, education and awareness of the facts and risks can help you to protect your family. Following are some tips to keep your children safe:

✔ Teach your child about touch. There is a difference between safe touch and touch that doesn't feel right. Make sure your toddler knows that no one should touch his private parts. Let your child know that he can say *no* to anybody who wants to touch him.

✔ Let your child show affection to friends and family members on his own terms. Don't make him kiss or hug someone.

✔ Let your child know early on that secrets are not okay. Most offenders try to trick children into thinking they can't tell anyone about what is happening because it is a secret. If your child knows that keeping secrets is not okay, he will know that something is wrong.

✔ Trust your child. Children don't lie about abuse. If your child tells you that some-one touched him and it didn't feel right, believe him!

✔ Remember that most perpetrators are people that you or your children are famil-iar with. The statistics show that it is not strangers we have to be aware of, but people who our children are taught to trust.

✔ Teach your child the proper names of body parts. You can begin by using the words *vagina* and *penis* during diaper changes. Having the right words to use makes communication between parents and children easier.

You can avoid power struggles with your toddler by choosing your battles wisely. For example, if your toddler wants to wear a winter hat in the summer, let her. However, if she wants to cross a busy street without holding your hand, that's obviously non-negotiable.

What if your toddler refuses a massage? We encourage you to respect what she says. Doing so sends her some clear messages:

✔ Her body is hers, and she has a say over who touches it. This is a very important message to give any child. The statistics on childhood sexual abuse indicate that 1 in 4 girls and 1 in 6 boys will be sexually abused by the age of 18. Perpetrators of sexual abuse are most often people that the child knows, not strangers. Teaching your toddler to say *no* to unwanted touch will decrease her vulnerability to being abused. For more tips, see the sidebar "How to protect your child from sexual abuse."

✔ You respect her feelings and her boundaries.

✔ You encourage her to be autonomous.

We also encourage you to respect your toddler when she specifically requests a massage. If you can't do it at that exact moment, tell her when you will be able to. Accommodating your toddler when she comes to you with such a request shows her that you are sensitive to her struggle with independence and dependence and that it's okay for her to have needs. Keep in mind that childhood needs that are met tend to go away. Needs that are not met are carried with us into adulthood.

Setting and respecting boundaries

Boundaries are what separate me from you; they simplify life and define expectations. Creating and setting boundaries for toddlers helps them be safe and lets them know what their limits are.

Here are some examples of common family boundaries:

✔ Knocking on a closed bedroom door before entering

✔ Asking permission before giving physical touch

✔ Prohibiting hitting and biting

Boundaries can also be rules and limits:

✔ "You must hold my hand while crossing the street."

✔ "You have to wear a coat in freezing weather."

✔ "You can't play with Daddy's laptop."

Babies and toddlers learn by watching how others behave. If you model clear and consistent boundaries with your partner and your other children, your younger children find out how to behave and have healthy relationships.

Here are some tips to help you be effective in setting boundaries:

✔ Be consistent. Toddlers and children get confused if your limits and rules are constantly changing.

✔ Be aware of your child's development. Knowing what she is capable of emotionally and physically lets you set realistic boundaries.

> ✔ Remember that setting boundaries is not about controlling your children. It's about keeping them safe and helping them learn self-discipline.

When massaging your older baby or toddler, you can set boundaries and let him know that you respect his by doing the following:

> ✔ Ask his permission to give him a massage.
>
> ✔ If your children are giving each other massages, make sure both are willing participants.
>
> ✔ Stop the massage if your child shows signs of overstimulation or is bored and looking for something else to do.
>
> ✔ Adhere to his requests. Sometimes toddlers have requests that may seem silly to us but are a way for them to express and practice their autonomy. For example, your toddler may be fine with you massaging his arms but refuses to let you touch his legs. This is a perfect opportunity for you to respect his boundaries.

Teaching discipline through massage

Massage gives you a consistent opportunity to create the kind of relationship your child needs in order to be receptive to gentle discipline. Here are some things that a child needs in order to respond favorably to loving guidance:

> ✔ Your child needs to trust you.
>
> ✔ He needs to recognize clear and consistent boundaries between you.
>
> ✔ He needs to learn how to communicate with you (both verbally and nonverbally).
>
> ✔ He needs to know that you are sensitive to his needs.

The word *discipline* literally means "to teach." Massaging your older baby or toddler actually helps you teach her about discipline, because massage helps children find out about boundaries, trust, and nonverbal communication. In fact, even a newborn or infant picks up lessons about discipline through massage.

Parents who massage and touch their children regularly become sensitive caretakers attuned to their children's needs. This type of parenting builds a relationship based on trust. Because you have responded to your children's needs with compassion and sensitivity, your babies grow up to respect (instead of fear) and count on your positive authority.

You create positive authority by doing the following:

✔ Not engaging in power struggles

✔ Setting appropriate limits and boundaries

✔ Disciplining your child with sensitivity and compassion

None of this means that you need to be a pushover. In fact, when you need to express your positive authority, it's best to be firm without being controlling or overbearing. Each time that you express positive authority, you strengthen trust and mutual respect with your children in a non-adversarial and cooperative way.

Continuing to massage your children enables you to stay attuned, sensitive, and aware of their changing needs. Your relationship will grow and evolve as they do.

For more information regarding discipline, we recommend the following books:

✔ *Natural Family Living: The Mother Magazine Guide to Parenting* by Peggy O'Mara (Pocket Books)

✔ *The Discipline Book: How to Have a Better-Behaved Child from Birth to Age Ten* by Martha and William Sears

Handling tantrums

The key to responding to temper tantrums appropriately begins with understanding why they occur. Toddlers typically have temper tantrums when they become overwhelmed with feelings that they do not know how to handle. Some things that trigger these intense feelings are being tired, hungry, frustrated, and angry.

Unfortunately, many times your toddler will have a tantrum in a public place, and you may feel overwhelmed with the responsibility of figuring out how best to handle the situation with people watching. Tantrums are very stressful for both you and your child.

Here are some suggestions to keep in mind for when a tantrum strikes:

✔ You need to try to remain as calm and objective as you can.

✔ You may need to literally hold your toddler so he doesn't hurt himself, or to carry him to somewhere safe and private.

✔ You don't want to just ignore the tantrum. Remember, your toddler is having a tantrum because he doesn't know how to handle intense emotions. Stay with him during the tantrum and do your best to remain loving. Use your intuition: Soothing words may help, but so may firm ones like "I know that you are angry and tired, but we have to finish shopping. If we don't finish, there won't be anything for dinner tonight."

✔ After your toddler has calmed down, spend some time talking with him and helping him find words for his feelings so you can both understand what happened.

✔ Because your toddler has experienced a lot of stress, you can help him release it by giving him a massage. Don't worry: You are not rewarding the tantrum by doing so. After he has calmed down and you have talked about what happened, giving him a massage reminds him that he does have the skills to calm himself down.

Chapter 10

Fitting Massage into Nap, Bath, and Diaper Time

In This Chapter

▶ Using massage before or after a nap

▶ Taking baths with your baby

▶ Making massage part of the diaper-changing routine

▶ Creating daily rituals

▶ Giving your baby a five-minute massage

*F*inding the right time to massage your baby is key to making the experience a success. In this chapter, we show you how to determine the best time based on several factors that may affect your massage. We demonstrate ways you can bring massage into your baby's life on a daily (or at least routine) basis, and we walk you through a five-minute massage. Finally, we have brainstormed about — and experimented with! — times and places you can massage your baby other than the usual culprits, and we share our insights with you.

Choosing the Right Time

To identify the right time to massage your baby, you need to take several factors into consideration:

✔ **Your baby's age:** We discuss this topic in the following section, "Deciding Whether to Stimulate or Not."

✔ **Your baby's tolerance level for stimulation:** We cover this topic in detail in the following section as well.

✔ **Your family's schedule:** If mornings are a hectic time for your family, for example, you may want to massage your baby in the late afternoon.

> ✔ **The goal of your massage:** Whether you want to stimulate your baby, put him to sleep, or address a common health ailment (which we discuss in Chapter 11) will help you determine the right time.
>
> ✔ **Any health or attachment issues your baby may have:** Chapters 11 and 12 cover issues that may affect when would be the best time for your baby to receive a massage.

Deciding Whether to Stimulate or Not

One of the first things you want to consider when deciding when to massage your baby is how your baby may respond to the stimulation of the massage. Age is a key factor: Some babies are very sensitive to stimulation, and some older babies and toddlers crave it.

Very young babies

In your baby's early weeks, it's best to keep the stimulation level to a minimum. If your baby is very sensitive to stimulation, just holding her may be enough in the beginning weeks, or you may use a limited massage routine with your baby's clothes on.

If you do use massage during your baby's first few weeks of life, here are some tips to keep in mind:

> ✔ If your young baby enjoys baths, try giving the massage before she takes a bath.
>
> ✔ If your young baby finds baths stressful, keep your massage and bathing experiences separate. For very sensitive babies, you may even want to bathe and massage on different days. (Later in this chapter, we offer tips on taking the stress out of the bathing experience.)
>
> ✔ You want to avoid giving a massage before naptime or bedtime because your baby may have trouble falling asleep.
>
> ✔ If you have a busy day of errands or visitors, you may want to skip the massage altogether because your own stress level may be too high.
>
> ✔ It's best to give the massage when the house is quiet and you are relaxed.
>
> ✔ You're better off skipping the massage altogether if finding the "right time" today is becoming stressful.

✔ You don't want to massage your baby during diaper changes until your baby is a little more experienced at receiving massages. Very young babies find diaper changes (and getting undressed) stressful. Adding stimulation on top of an already stimulating and stressful situation may be just too much.

More experienced babies

After you've been giving your baby massages for a while — one to three months — you won't have to be so careful about her stimulation level. If she hasn't already, she'll soon begin to relax during a massage, regardless of what time of day it is.

Keep in mind that relaxed doesn't necessarily mean sleepy. Your baby may be relaxed yet alert and wanting to play after a massage. On the other hand, with the right technique, you can put your relaxed baby to sleep in no time by using massage.

If you are not worried about stimulating your baby too much, here are some tips to keep in mind:

✔ You can massage your baby throughout the day by focusing on different parts of his body during each diaper change.

✔ You can start off a busy day with a bath followed by a massage. Your baby will be relaxed and alert, making the day easier for both of you.

✔ It's possible to use a bath and massage to cure the boredom blues for both of you!

Massaging Baby Before or After Nap

You are the best judge of whether to massage your baby before or after he takes a nap, based on his potential for stimulation. In this section, we help you determine if your baby is getting enough sleep and how you can help him get more if he has trouble napping. Also, if you choose to massage him immediately prior to or after a nap, we offer some suggestions for which massage techniques to use.

Studies conducted by the Touch Research Institute in 2001 indicate that babies who receive a massage by a parent before going to sleep fall asleep with less difficulty and have better sleep quality.

When will my baby sleep through the night?

This may be the question parents most frequently ask of doctors and other parents. The truth is that when babies are young, "sleeping through the night" really means sleeping for about a five-hour stretch. Babies simply aren't wired to sleep for much longer at one time. They have shorter sleep cycles than adults and wake repeatedly through the night. Sleep problems often arise for the parents because some babies have difficulty falling back to sleep.

You can try a variety of methods and follow many different philosophies to help your baby fall back asleep. We are advocates of the gentle approach to parenting your baby back to sleep. Your coauthor Joanne has used massage to successfully help her daughter Ava get back to sleep. On the few occasions that Ava woke up in the middle of the night wanting to play, giving her a massage proved tremendously helpful in coaxing her to go back to sleep.

You can find more gentle approaches to helping your baby sleep in *The Baby Book* by William and Martha Sears and *The No-Cry Sleep Solution: Gentle Ways to Help Your Baby Sleep Through the Night* by Elizabeth Pantley (Contemporary Books).

Knowing how much sleep to expect

You can determine how much sleep your baby should be getting by his age. Below are the ranges of sleep that babies need, on average, at certain ages:

- Birth to 3 months: 15 to 18 hours per day
- 3 to 6 months: 13 to 16 hours a day
- 6 months to 2 years: 12 to 14 hours a day

Realizing the importance of naps

You want to encourage your baby to nap during the day so that the quality of her nighttime sleep is better. Babies who skip naps become overly tired and have a difficult time falling and staying asleep.

Newborns nap frequently; they typically sleep after every feeding, which means every two to four hours (depending on your baby and whether you are using formula or breastfeeding). As your baby grows older, she needs less frequent naps.

Around 6 to 9 months of age, your baby will probably settle into a routine of taking two naps per day: one in the morning and one in the afternoon. Sometime around 12 months, she may begin to have only one longer nap per day, perhaps in the early afternoon.

Timing your massage right

If you want to give your baby a pre-nap massage, be sure to time it right. It doesn't take long for your baby to develop a general routine: You'll begin to notice that he typically takes naps around the same time every day, and you can look for the following signs that he's getting sleepy:

- ✔ He becomes fussy.
- ✔ He rubs his eyes.
- ✔ He stares off into space.
- ✔ He's easily frustrated.

You want to plan your massage in advance so that the massage isn't pushing him past his nap time, which may actually keep him awake. Instead, use the massage to gently lead him into sleep.

We don't recommend that you give your baby a massage before every nap. He may become accustomed to falling asleep this way and begin to rely on a massage to sleep.

Sometimes babies refuse to nap. If yours does, you may need to establish a routine for him. For example, around the time he should be napping, begin a massage to relax him. At other times, use other methods to induce sleep such as rocking him, wearing him in a sling, or taking him for a walk in the stroller.

It's easy to take the power struggle out of nap time. Actions like massaging your baby or wearing him in a sling let him fall asleep naturally.

Giving a great massage before a nap

Certain techniques are naturally more soothing to babies than others, and in this section we've put together some techniques from Chapters 5, 6, and 7 that we think are great to use before naptime.

For a massage before naptime, use only strokes that move in a downward direction. Strokes that move up (toward the heart) are too stimulating.

The sequence of techniques that we recommend in this section are for babies who have been receiving massage regularly for some time and are able to tolerate it.

The Sleeper

Even for a baby experienced at receiving massages, there are a lot of techniques in this sequence. Feel free to omit some if time and your baby's tolerance level do not allow all of them.

1. **Massage both the front and back side of the legs using the following techniques (see Chapters 5 and 7):**
   - The Taffy Pull
   - Thumb Circles
   - Raking

2. **Massage the belly using the following techniques (see Chapter 5):**
   - The Water Wheel
   - The Open Book Stroke

3. **Massage the buttocks using the Large Bottom Stroke (see Chapter 7).**

4. **Massage the back using the Long Effleurage Stroke (see Chapter 7).**

5. **Massage the hands using the following strokes (see Chapter 5):**
   - Alternating Hands
   - Hand stroking
   - Finger stroking

6. **Massage the neck and shoulders using Long Strokes (see Chapter 7).**

7. **Massage the face using the following techniques (see Chapter 6):**
   - Small Circles
   - Tapping the Jaw Line

The Little Sleeper

Here is a pre-nap massage sequence for your little one who is just beginning to receive massages and may be easily stimulated.

Use this sequence on the front side of the body only. All these techniques are shown in Chapter 5.

1. **Massage the legs using the following techniques:**
   - The Taffy Pull
   - Ankles Away
2. **Massage the feet using This Little Piggy.**
3. **Massage the arms using the following strokes:**
   - Alternating Hands
   - Finger stroking

The abdomen and chest are high stimulation areas. We have purposefully left these parts of the body out of the above massage sequences.

Giving a great massage after a nap

After a nap is a perfect time to use some techniques that stimulate your baby. In this section we show some sequences to try.

One difference between a massage that's stimulating and one that isn't is the use of *petrissage strokes* — kneading strokes that are used on loose, heavy musculature tissue. You can find out more about petrissage strokes in the "Kneading Dough" section in Chapter 5.

Another key to creating a massage that's stimulating is using some of your strokes in an upward direction: moving them toward your baby's head.

Let's Go!

This sequence creates an ideal massage for older babies who have had a lot of massages and have a high tolerance for stimulation. However, you always have to keep in mind that not all babies are the same: Your baby may love all the techniques, become bored halfway through, or even become too stimulated. Keep an eye out for signs that your baby has had enough.

In this list of techniques, we have indicated that some are good to use in both upward and downward strokes.

1. **Massage the front of the legs using the following techniques (see Chapter 5):**
   - The Taffy Pull
   - Either Kneading Dough (using downward and upward strokes) or Thumb Circles (using downward and upward strokes)
2. **Massage the feet using This Little Piggy (see Chapter 5).**

3. **Massage the front side of the legs using Raking (see Chapter 5).**

4. **Massage the belly using the following techniques (see Chapter 5):**

   - Thumbs to Sides

   - Sun and Moon stroke

5. **Massage the chest and shoulders using the Butterfly Stroke (see Chapter 5).**

6. **Massage the arms and hands using the following techniques (see Chapter 5):**

   - The "C" Stroke

   - Hand stroking

7. **Massage the back side of the legs using Kneading Dough or Thumb Circles using upward and downward strokes (see Chapter 7).**

8. **Massage the buttocks using the following techniques (see Chapter 7):**

   - Alternating Thumbs

   - Finger stroking

9. **Massage the back using the following techniques (see Chapter 7):**

   - The Long Effleurage Stroke

   - Back and Forth (moving upward and downward)

   - Swooping (moving upward and downward)

Let's Go Jr.

If the previous sequence seems like too much for your little one, here is a sequence that is just stimulating enough for most babies.

To reduce the stimulation level further, work only the front or back side of the body at one time. You can even split the massage between naps. For example, after your baby wakes from her morning nap, massage the front side of her body. Save the back side for when she wakes from her afternoon nap.

1. **Massage the front of the legs and feet using the following techniques (see Chapter 5):**

   - The Taffy Pull (using upward and downward strokes)

   - Thumb Circles (using downward strokes only)

   - This Little Piggy

2. **Massage the belly using The Water Wheel (see Chapter 5).**

3. **Massage the chest and shoulders using the Open Book Stroke (see Chapter 5).**

4. **Massage the arms and hands using the following techniques (see Chapter 5):**

   - Alternating Hands

   - Finger stroking

5. **Massage the back of the legs using Thumb Circles in downward strokes only (see Chapter 7).**

6. **Massage the buttocks using Alternating Thumbs (see Chapter 7).**

7. **Massage the back using the following techniques (see Chapter 7):**

   - The Sacral Stroke

   - Swooping

   - Raking

If you have very little time but want to give your baby a quickie massage, just use the Raking technique in both downward and upward movements. You can even do this with your baby's clothes on.

Sudden infant death syndrome (SIDS)

Most new parents are keenly aware that SIDS is an as-yet unexplained cause of death in babies 12 months and under. Here's how you can reduce the risk of losing your baby to SIDS:

✔ Always place your baby on his or her back to sleep.

✔ Breastfeed. (Frequent feedings increase the amount of contact during the night between you and your baby, reducing the risk of SIDS.)

✔ Avoid keeping toys and stuffed animals in the crib.

✔ Don't let anyone smoke around your baby.

✔ Don't use fluffy comforters or blankets in your baby's crib.

✔ Consider co-sleeping with your baby (see Chapter 3).

✔ Make sure that your baby doesn't get overheated during sleep.

You can find more information on SIDS at the National SIDS/Infant Death Resource Center's Web site (www.sidscenter.org).

Waking your baby gently with massage

"Never wake a sleeping baby" is usually good advice. However, at times you're going to have to wake your baby to take him to the sitter or to a "Mommy (or Daddy) and Me" class. What better way to wake your little one than with a massage?

Babies sleep the safest on their backs (see the sidebar on "Sudden infant death syndrome [SIDS]"). We're assuming that your baby is on his back as you begin this massage.

Here are the steps to take to gently wake your baby:

1. **While he is sleeping, greet your little one with sweet and soothing words while you gently place your hands on his chest and hold them there for a moment or two.**

2. **Slowly and gently, use the Raking technique described in Chapter 5 down the length of your baby's entire body.** Repeat this technique three to five times.

3. **Make sure that you have a loving smile on your face and gaze softly into your baby's eyes when he begins to wake up and see you.**

   If your baby tends to cry when he wakes up, stop here and pick him up. (Chances are that he will stop crying when he wakes if this massage is what he has to look forward to!)

4. **If your baby likes to have his face touched, use the Small Circles and Circling the Eyes techniques shown in Chapter 6.**

5. **Use the Open Book Stroke shown in Chapter 6 on your baby's forehead.**

6. **Finish with a hug!**

Taking Baby in the Bath with You

Bathing with your baby is a convenient way for you to mix play, skin-on-skin contact, warmth, and massage all at once. In this section, we show you how to do so in ways that are safe and enjoyable for both of you.

Playing it safe

Here are some tips to help you make bathing with your baby safe:

✔ Always check the water temperature before you bring your baby into the tub.

✔ Plan ahead for the bath and have everything you need nearby: shampoo, washcloth, car/infant seat (to place your baby in while you get in and out of the tub), towels (one for you, too!), soap, and tub toys.

If you plan to give your baby an after-bath massage (which we discuss in upcoming sections), place a diaper and change of clothes near where you will be giving the massage, such as near the changing table.

✔ If you're bathing with a newborn, have your partner or a helper nearby.

✔ Check the perimeter ledge of the tub beforehand and make sure that everything your little one can reach with her hands is safe. (Move those razors!)

✔ Keep in mind how slippery your little one will be when she's soaped up!

Bathing with a newborn

A baby's first bath can be very stressful: Your baby may be terrified of being placed in a small tub of water, and you may feel like a bad parent for making him cry. You may be able to skip the stress by taking your baby in the bath with you. Most newborns love this experience; the combination of feeling the warm water and hearing your heartbeat and voice makes your baby feel as if he is back in the womb.

Be sure you wait until your baby's umbilical cord falls off before giving him a full bath. If you are unsure about this, ask your family doctor or pediatrician. And keep in mind that newborns need to be bathed only once or twice a week.

The first couple of times you bring your newborn in the bath with you can be a little nerve-racking because of the combination of your baby's slippery, soapy skin and lack of head control. But with practice, you can make the experience comfortable and fun. (Your co-author Joanne can attest: She's been taking her daughter in the bath with her since she was just a couple of weeks old.) Here are some tips to make it a safe and pleasurable experience for both of you:

- ✔ For your first couple of baths, have someone with you who can help you bring your baby in and out of the tub and soap him up.

- ✔ Fill the tub approximately two-thirds full before you get in, and check that the temperature is warm but not too hot.

Be sure to watch the water level when your baby is placed on your chest. If it's too close to his mouth and nose, let some water out.

- ✔ Keep an infant or car seat near the tub, and place your baby's towel inside the seat. Before you get in the bath, put your baby in the seat.

- ✔ Get in the tub first by yourself. If you're taking your first bath since giving birth, go ahead and take a few minutes by yourself before bringing your baby in with you. You will really appreciate the break!

- ✔ Have your partner (or helper) slowly and gently place your baby chest-down on top of your chest.

Your baby responds to your emotions. If you are calm and relaxed, your baby will be, too.

- ✔ Gently hold your baby and feel him relax and melt into your skin.

- ✔ Have your partner or helper soap up a soft baby's washcloth and gently wash your baby. Keep a squirt bottle nearby to help rinse your baby off.

In the early days, it may be difficult to wash the front side of your baby's body. You can wash his belly on the changing table with a sponge bath if necessary.

- ✔ Spend a few minutes just holding your little one and rubbing his back.

- ✔ When it's time to get out of the bath, have your helper or partner take the baby out first and immediately place him in the car seat. Wrap the towel around him (like a cocoon) to keep him warm.

Some people recommend breastfeeding during the bath. It is a very pleasurable experience for your baby to be nursed and surrounded by warm water. However, most newborns' elimination process occurs immediately following a feeding, so nursing in the bathtub may not be so pleasurable for you!

Giving your newborn an after-bath massage

When you have finished bathing with your baby, you can take her to a flat surface (still wrapped in the towel) and give her a gentle massage. Use the towel to keep the parts of her body that are not being massaged covered.

Because you are massaging a newborn, use downward strokes on the front side of the body only and keep the length of your massage short. Also, speak softly and sweetly to your baby throughout the massage, and be sure to make a lot of eye contact.

Here are the steps involved in a great after-bath massage:

1. **Uncover one leg at a time from the towel, and use The Taffy Pull and This Little Piggy strokes shown in Chapter 5.**

2. **Take one arm out from under the towel at a time, and use the Alternating Hands technique we show in Chapter 5.**

You're finished! This short massage is enough stimulation for most newborns.

Keep a clean diaper and fresh clothes nearby so when you are finished with the massage you can quickly diaper and outfit your baby.

Bathing with your older baby

When your baby begins to gain some head control, you can bring eye contact and play into your bath. By bending your knees and placing your baby with her back against your thighs, you and she are in a good position to give and receive smiles, laughter, and love. You can also wash her belly!

Here are some tips to make bathing with your older baby fun and safe:

✔ Place a car/infant seat (with your baby's towel inside) next to the tub.

✔ Put your baby in the car/infant seat, and after you are in the tub, reach over the side and pick her up. You will be able to put her back in the car/infant seat the same way after you've finished bathing.

✔ Have some brightly colored floating toys in the tub for her to play with. Encourage splashing!

✔ If your baby is 6 months or older, place him or her in a seated position on your extended legs, facing out. This will make your baby feel like a big boy or girl!

✔ Finish the bath chest-to-chest with your baby. Let her feel her legs and arms floating, and watch her relax.

Giving your older baby an after-bath massage

The type of massage you give your older baby after his bath will depend on his experience with massage and whether you would like to stimulate him or put him to sleep. See the sections "Giving a great massage before a nap" and "Giving a great massage after a nap" earlier in this chapter for ideas. Be sure to use your baby's towel to keep him warm during the massage.

We encourage you to follow your baby's cues and your instincts. With an older baby, you can begin to experiment with different techniques and see how he responds.

 Try only two or three new strokes at any time with your baby. By doing so, you'll have an easier time getting a feel for which ones your baby likes and dislikes.

Bringing Massage to the Changing Table

Let's face it: There is going to be a lot of diaper changing in your future — newborns typically urinate every hour and can have bowel movements five to ten times a day. You may as well make diaper changing a fun experience for you and your baby! In this section, we show you how.

Changing your newborn

For newborns, a diaper change is a stressful thing. Everything is brand new to them, and they don't understand why every hour or so they are undressed, moved around, wiped, and dressed again. You can help make diaper changing a better experience for your newborn by practicing these tips:

✔ Make sure you have everything you need nearby: diapers, wipes, diaper rash cream, and a clean outfit in case of a leak.

✔ Move slowly and gently and use a calm, soothing voice.

If you are anxious about changing a newborn and are experiencing stress, your newborn will feel it and become stressed, too.

✔ Use a baby wipe warmer: Your newborn will show her appreciation by crying less.

✔ Keep some stuffed animals and musical toys nearby so you can play with your newborn during or after the diaper change.

✔ Sing nursery rhymes.

✔ Incorporate massage into the process, as your baby tolerates.

Bringing massage to the changing table with a newborn is easy. We make it even easier for you by listing here the techniques from Chapter 5 that are appropriate for a newborn.

Use only one or two techniques at a time — using downward strokes only — for your newborn. You can add more as her tolerance for stimulation is increased. Here are the strokes to try:

✔ The Taffy Pull

✔ Ankles Away

✔ This Little Piggy

✔ Raking

✔ Alternating Hands

✔ The "C" Stroke

✔ Thumb Circles

✔ Hands on Hands

✔ Finger stroking

It's a good idea to try these strokes out on your baby first with his clothes on, so wait to begin the massage until after you have finished changing his diaper (and outfit, if necessary). With the exception of This Little Piggy, any of the above strokes can be done on your newborn with his clothes on.

You can also try to include massaging your baby's face while on the changing table. He may not like this at all at first, so be patient; you can always use these strokes later on. Here are some strokes from Chapter 6 to try:

✔ Small Circles

✔ The Open Book Stroke (first variation)

✔ The Temple Stroke

Changing your older baby

By now you and your baby have shared many diaper changes together. To continue making diaper changes a good time for contact and bonding, plus to relieve boredom, here are some tips:

✔ Babies love to practice their new skills. When your baby is able to sit up, let her do so on the changing table while you keep her stable with one hand. Use this opportunity to massage her back while you acknowledge what a big girl she is.

✔ Warm up your baby's legs for standing with the following strokes (see Chapters 5 and 7):

• The Taffy Pull

• Kneading Dough

• Squeeze and Twist

When you are finished with these strokes, lay her on her back on the floor (so you avoid getting your baby used to standing on the changing table), grab onto her wrists, and gently pull her up to standing. Tell her what a big girl she is.

✔ Help your toddler learn names for his different body parts by making it a game. Ask him: "Where is your arm?" When he shows you, reward him with a stroke such as Alternating Hands or the "C" Stroke (see Chapter 5).

Making Daily Massage Routine

If you've read this whole chapter, you should have some good ideas on how to massage your baby daily. There are plenty of opportunities for massage around naps, baths, and diaper changes. In this section we show you how to use massage to create rituals with your baby, plus we walk you through a five-minute massage you can do anytime.

Creating rituals

Rituals help you to create tradition in your family, as well as to establish consistency and routines for your children. Your baby will quickly become familiar with your routines and come to count on rituals to help her feel secure, to know what's coming next, and to learn new things.

Keep two things in mind when creating rituals:

✓ Rituals are repetitive.

✓ Rituals are positive: They make your baby feel good.

By including massage in your routine, you are creating a ritual with your baby that makes her feel good. Here are some ways you can make massage a ritual in your family:

✓ Give your baby a massage after every bath.

✓ Whenever your baby achieves a developmental milestone, celebrate with enthusiasm and a massage.

✓ Make massage part of your nighttime sleep ritual.

✓ Make changing diapers fun for you and your baby by including singing, games, and a massage.

Giving a five-minute massage

Whenever you have five free minutes and want to make it great quality time for you and your baby, try this massage sequence. You can position your baby on a bed, a changing table, or your lap.

1. **Massage the front side of the legs using the following techniques (see Chapter 5):**

   • The Taffy Pull

   • Kneading Dough

2. **Massage the belly using the Sun and Moon technique (see Chapter 5).**

3. **Massage the chest using The Open Book Stroke (see Chapter 5).**

4. **Massage the arms and hands using the following techniques (see Chapter 5):**

   • Alternating Hands

   • Hand stroking

   • Finger stroking

5. **Massage the back side of the legs using Kneading Dough (see Chapter 7).**

6. **Massage the buttocks using the Large Bottom Stroke** (see Chapter 7).

7. **Massage the back using Swooping (see Chapter 7).**

8. **Massage the face using the Open Book Stroke (first variation; see Chapter 6).**

Identifying More Good Times and Places for Massage

There are so many times and places to massage your baby that we thought we would give you just a few more ideas. Let these spark your own creativity:

✔ Take your baby to the park for a picnic, spread out a blanket, and begin your massage.

✔ Massage your baby while waiting in the doctor's office. You can do this by laying your baby sideways on your lap (see Figure 7-1 in Chapter 7).

✔ Massage your baby on an airplane. For an older baby, let him sit on your lap, facing out. With one hand, you can massage his back.

✔ Place your baby on your lap sideways and massage her back while you are talking on the phone.

✔ If your baby begins to fuss in a restaurant, take him out of the highchair, place him on your lap, and massage his back.

✔ If you are waiting in a long line in a supermarket, keep your baby seated and buckled safely in the cart, and use Hands on Hands and Finger stroking (see Chapter 5) to keep her busy.

✔ When you wear your baby in a sling, use one hand to do the Circling the Eyes stroke (see Chapter 6) and the Open Book Stroke (see Chapter 5).

✔ If you are traveling a long distance in a car, sit in the back with your baby and massage his legs, arms, and face while he stays safely in the car seat.

Part IV
Easing Health Problems with Massage

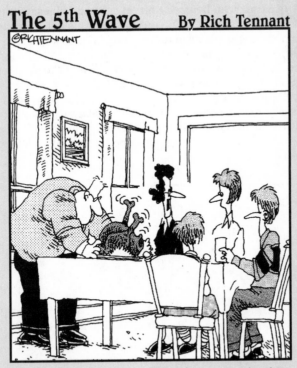

The 5th Wave   By Rich Tennant

"If massaging the baby relaxes him so much, think
how tender it'll make the turkey."

In this part . . .

Massage can be used to treat common illnesses and health problems in your baby. In this part, we show you how to use massage to treat conditions like colic, asthma, and congestion. We also explain why attachment is crucial and how you can use massage and touch to help you bond with an adopted or foster baby. Babies with developmental delays have special needs for touch and massage that we cover here as well. Finally, we show you how to use massage and touch techniques to help babies who are addicted to drugs, exposed to alcohol, or affected by HIV.

Chapter 11

Massage for Common Ailments and Problems

In This Chapter

▶ Using abdominal strokes to relieve constipation

▶ Addressing colic and asthma with massage

▶ Soothing the pain of teething

▶ Clearing congestion

▶ Calming the fussy baby

▶ Treating dry skin

At one time or another, most babies experience constipation, congestion, dry skin, or fussiness. And all babies experience teething, of course. Massage is an easy and effective way to help your baby feel better as he deals with these common ailments and developmental milestones.

In the case of colic or having a high need baby, we believe that taking care of yourself is just as important to your family's health as taking care of your little one. For this reason, in this chapter we also offer ideas on how you can find support and take steps to care for yourself until you and your baby get past these stressful stages.

 Always check with your pediatrician or family practice doctor if you are using massage to treat a health issue, to be sure there aren't any contraindications.

Relieving Constipation

Constipation in infants and babies typically means having stools that are hard, dry, infrequent, and sometimes painful. As we explain in this section, babies who are exclusively breastfed don't tend to have this problem; babies who become constipated are usually formula-fed, just beginning to eat solids, or both.

Bypassing the problem with breastfeeding

Babies who are breastfed exclusively don't usually become constipated because breast milk is easily digested. Breastfed babies also have some other advantages when it comes to digestion:

- ✔ Breastfed babies have bacteria in their intestines that break down proteins and create softer stool.

- ✔ Breastfed babies also have higher levels of the hormone motilin than formula-fed babies. Motilin helps keep the bowels moving.

Recognizing discomfort in formula-fed babies

Formula-fed babies have a higher risk of constipation than breastfed babies because formula is not as easily digested as breast milk. Also, allergies to formula can cause constipation. Here are some signs that your baby may be allergic to formula:

- ✔ Your baby continues to be fussy after a feeding.

- ✔ Her belly is distended, and she is gassy.

- ✔ She has a red rectum that diaper rash cream won't clear up.

- ✔ She spits up frequently.

- ✔ Her bowel movements tend to be either very hard or watery.

Spitting up, fussiness, and gas may also be signs that your baby is getting too much formula in one feeding.

Saving solids until baby is ready

Some babies are introduced to solids at an early age, before their digestive systems are fully formed. Sometimes solids can create dehydration as your baby's digestive system becomes used to digesting a particular food.

Most babies are ready to start solid foods sometime around the age of 6 months, although each baby is slightly different. Talk with your pediatrician about the right time and way to introduce solids to your baby, and when you do, pay careful attention to any changes in his stools. If he starts to experience constipation when solids are introduced to his diet, he may not be ready for them yet.

Counteracting constipation

Several massage techniques that we demonstrate in Chapter 5 are effective in alleviating constipation:

- ✔ The Water Wheel
- ✔ Thumbs to Sides
- ✔ Sun and Moon
- ✔ I Love You

Try giving your baby a belly massage for constipation after she takes a warm bath.

Always use strokes in a clockwise direction on the abdomen. And be sure to use a little pressure to avoid the tickle response!

In addition to using these massage techniques, you can incorporate the following tips to keep your baby's bowels moving:

- ✔ Place your baby on his belly on your knee. The pressure from this position will help move the gas or stool out of his intestinal tract.
- ✔ Place your baby lying face down with his belly on your forearm and his head near your elbow. Put pressure on his belly with your arm and hand (visualize how a football player cradles his football). Rub his sacrum with your other hand. (If you are unsure where the sacrum is, take a look at Figure 7-12 in Chapter 7.)
- ✔ Place your baby on your chest or over your shoulder and massage his sacrum and lower back.
- ✔ While your baby is on his back, imagine a clock on his belly. Use your fingertips to make tiny clockwise circles that being at 7:00 and work around to 5:00.

The above techniques can all be done while your baby's clothes are on.

Recognizing and Responding to Colic

Approximately 25 percent of babies experience *colic* — a condition that causes babies to cry inconsolably for at least three hours a day at least three days a week. Keep in mind that this is the *minimum* amount of crying for a diagnosis; some babies cry for hours on end with no apparent reason — they simply will not stop.

If your baby has colic, he may cry, scream, and kick for hours. He may arch his back and tighten his stomach. He seems like he is in a lot of pain, and you can't find the cause of it. Needless to say, colic is stressful for the whole family.

The best news we can offer is that most cases of colic disappear somewhere around 3 to 4 months of age. Hang in there!

Looking for causes of colic

The truth is that no one really knows what causes colic. Following are some common theories:

- ✔ An immature digestive system

- ✔ Emotional stress

- ✔ An immature nervous system

- ✔ Food allergies — for example, if a breastfeeding mother is drinking cow's milk and eating dairy products, or if an infant is drinking formula (either milk- or soy-based)

- ✔ Your baby's temperament

- ✔ Gastroesophageal reflux disease (GERD) — a condition that affects babies and adults alike and is commonly called *reflux*

We believe that colic is probably caused by a combination of these factors.

Massaging to ease colic

Regular abdominal massage may lower the frequency and severity of your baby's colic episodes. You can use any of the belly massages we show in Chapter 5 (which are listed in the "Counteracting constipation" section earlier in this chapter) to help prevent an episode of colic. These techniques help you stimulate your baby's colon and push gas and stool through the intestinal tract.

Here are some additional massage, exercise, and holding techniques you can use during a colic attack:

✔ Hold your baby in the football hold. Place your baby lying face down with his belly on your forearm and his head near your elbow. Put pressure on his belly with your arm and hand (visualize how a football player cradles his football). Rub his sacrum with your other hand.

✔ Place your baby on his back, and bring both knees to his chest by bending his legs. Your hands are on the outside of your baby's knees. Hold his knees on his chest for a few seconds.

You can also do this technique one leg at a time.

✔ Follow the instructions in the previous bullet and, with both legs together, circle your baby's knees clockwise (in the direction of the colon).

Offering your baby additional relief

Here are some other ways that you can try to comfort your baby during an episode of colic:

✔ Wear your baby in a sling (see Chapter 1).

✔ Run the vacuum.

✔ Swaddle your baby (see Chapter 3).

✔ Take your baby for a ride in the car.

✔ Use an infant swing or an Amby Baby Motion Bed (see www.AmbyBaby.com).

✔ Take a warm bath with your baby (see Chapter 10).

✔ Try feeding your baby more slowly (and possibly less) during each feeding.

Try to alternate comfort measures. For example, you may wear your baby in a sling for a while, then take a warm bath together, and then go for a ride in the car.

We know how stressful colic can be, but we do not recommend letting your baby cry it out. If you have tried everything you can think of to calm him and your baby is still crying, simply hold him and speak soothingly throughout the episode. If your frustration level has peaked, ask your partner, your friends, and your family for help. Being held while crying is a much different and better experience for a baby than being left alone in a crib.

What's the risk of letting your baby cry it out? Your baby will not learn important self-soothing skills, and unfortunately he may learn that his needs will not be met and his environment is not safe. He may also learn to shut down his feelings.

No matter how frustrated you may get, do not ever shake your baby. A baby can die or suffer permanent brain damage after being shaken. If you are overwhelmed and start to feel yourself getting angry at your baby, place him in a safe place (such as his crib or playpen) and go into another room to give yourself time to calm down. Practicing the breathing techniques we show you in Chapters 2 and 4 can help as well.

Easing your own stress

Colic is most definitely a family affair. For this reason, we want to offer some suggestions on how to cope so the stress doesn't overwhelm you:

- ✔ Take a break. Find a way to spend at least an hour away from your baby each day.

- ✔ Get support. Locate other parents of colicky babies — perhaps through La Leche League meetings, Mommy and Me classes, or other local groups that bring new parents together. If you don't know where to look for this type of organization, contact the hospital where you delivered your baby and ask for help finding a support group.

- ✔ If you're not able to find a support group that meets your needs, at least find one person you can share your feelings of frustration with.

- ✔ Let someone give *you* a massage!

- ✔ Remind yourself not to take your baby's crying personally — it is absolutely not a reflection of your parenting abilities.

Breathing Easy: Coping with Asthma

Asthma is a chronic condition where airways become inflamed and filled with mucus that causes wheezing and difficulty breathing. If your baby has an asthma attack, she coughs and her lungs spasm to remove the mucus.

The most common type of asthma is caused by allergies. When exposed to an allergen (like mold or pollen), the body creates an antibody that releases a chemical substance called a *mediator*. Mediators cause the airways to become inflamed, which results in asthma symptoms.

Reducing asthma triggers

You may not be able to prevent your baby from getting asthma, but you can help her by removing some of things in your home environment that may trigger it. Here are some things you can do:

✔ Never smoke near your baby.

✔ Limit her exposure to dust.

✔ If you are a breastfeeding mother, avoid eating foods that many people are allergic to, such as eggs, nuts, and shellfish.

✔ Do not use a wood stove or fireplace.

✔ Monitor your baby's stress level. Stress can create anxiety symptoms like shortness of breath, which can trigger an asthma attack or make a current attack feel worse.

It typically takes six months of exposure to a potential allergen for an allergy to show up. That's why babies 6 months and older may begin to show allergies to pets or particular foods. Children don't get seasonal allergies until around the age of 4 or 5.

Seeing signs of asthma

Diagnosing asthma in very young babies can be difficult, so many infants' asthma goes undiagnosed. Following are some symptoms that your baby may display if he has asthma:

✔ Frequent chest colds

✔ A rattly cough

✔ Difficulty feeding

✔ Rapid breathing

✔ A whistling or wheezing noise when exhaling

✔ Shortness of breath

If you are at all concerned that your baby may have asthma, contact your pediatrician and describe exactly the types of symptoms your baby is experiencing. It's crucial to have asthma diagnosed as soon as possible.

Recognizing asthma attacks

Asthma attacks are frightening for both parents and babies. When your baby is having difficulty breathing, neither of you feels like you have any control over the situation.

Typically, doctors classify asthma attacks in three categories:

- ✓ **Mild:** Your baby's breathing is affected; she has some wheezing, coughing, and shortness of breath. She is alert, and her skin color is normal.

- ✓ **Moderate:** Your baby's skin becomes pale, and she experiences more wheezing, whistling, and shortness of breath than in a mild asthma attack. She is still alert.

- ✓ **Severe:** Breathing is extremely difficult. Wheezing and coughing are severe, and your baby is no longer alert — she may be very drowsy. Her skin color may be blue or extremely pale.

Talk with your pediatrician about the steps you should take during an asthma attack; she will help you create an action plan.

Massaging for asthma

To help alleviate the symptoms of asthma, you want to focus on massaging your baby's upper chest. The chest-opening techniques that we show you in Chapter 5 are appropriate to use during mild asthma attacks and are good preventative care to prevent attacks from occurring:

- ✓ The Heart Stroke
- ✓ The Open Book Stroke
- ✓ The Butterfly Stroke

If your baby is having a moderate or severe asthma attack, we recommend calling your healthcare provider. Giving your baby a relaxing massage after the asthma attack can help reduce the effects of the stressful attack.

Ouch! Helping Teething Pain

Sharp tiny teeth poking through your baby's gums can cause a lot of pain. Some babies seem to suffer tremendously during teething, while others experience only mild discomfort. In either case, knowing how to respond to your baby's pain begins with identifying whether your baby is truly teething or not.

Anticipating their arrival

Your baby actually starts teething while still in the womb; that's when tooth buds (all 20 of them) begin to form under the gum. But a baby's teeth usually don't cut through the gum until at least several months after birth.

You can expect to see signs of teething and your baby's first teeth erupt around 6 months of age. But keep in mind that 6 months is just an approximation; some babies cut their first tooth at 3 months (or even earlier)!

Typically, the first teeth you see are the upper and lower incisors, followed by the first molars, the canine teeth, and then your baby's 2-year molars.

Your child's permanent teeth won't be ready to come in until somewhere around the age of 6.

Recognizing signs of teething

Many signs can point to the fact that your baby is teething. Here are some of them:

- ✔ She drools a lot — so much that she may need to wear a bib. The excessive drooling may cause diarrhea or loose stools.

- ✔ She is very fussy.

- ✔ She wants to chew on her toys (and anything else she can get her hands and mouth on).

- ✔ She pulls on her ears.

- ✔ She may have a slight fever.

- ✔ She has a dry cough.

- ✔ She may suddenly cry out in pain.

- ✔ She may wake up at night more frequently than normal.

- ✔ She may start biting.

If you suspect that teeth are on their way, use the finger test: Make sure your finger is very clean, and rub it along your baby's gums. If a tooth is twisting its way through, you will feel it!

Massaging to ease the pain

Keep in mind that your baby's gums, mouth, and facial muscles may be very sensitive during teething. Try one or two of the following techniques and note your baby's response and sensitivity level. If he responds well, continue. If not, try one of the other suggestions we offer later in this section.

Massage techniques that focus on your baby's face, forehead, and neck are appropriate when focusing on teething pain; each of these areas is prone to the effects of teething stress. Try any of the following techniques, which we show you in Chapter 6:

- ✔ Ears to Chin
- ✔ Small Circles
- ✔ Tapping the Jaw Line
- ✔ The Smile Stroke
- ✔ Circling the Eyes
- ✔ The Open Book Stroke
- ✔ Big Circles
- ✔ The Temple Stroke
- ✔ The Ear Stroke
- ✔ Chinny Chin Chin
- ✔ Scooping

Breastfeeding and teething

Some breastfeeding moms think they need to stop nursing when their babies begin teething. The truth is that you can continue to nurse even if your baby has a full set of teeth! If your baby is latched onto your breast correctly, he cannot bite while he's nursing because his tongue covers his gums between his lower teeth and your breast.

It is those brief moments just before and just after nursing that you need to look out for. If your baby does bite you, your startle reaction may be enough to stop him from doing it again. But be sure not to pull your baby away quickly — you may really hurt yourself if he latches on. Instead, pull your baby close to you, which prevents him from breathing through his nose momentarily and forces him to de-latch himself. You can also de-latch him by inserting your pinky finger into your baby's mouth to release the suction.

Here are some other ways you can help your baby through teething by using touch:

✔ Let your baby gnaw and chomp away on your clean finger.

✔ Use a clean finger to push down gently on your baby's gums to help relieve some of the pressure.

✔ Hold and cuddle with your baby a lot.

✔ Wear him in a sling.

✔ Consider co-sleeping (see Chapter 3) because you are better able to comfort your baby during the night.

Offering additional relief

Together with massage and touch, you can also use some of the tried-and-true methods of helping teething pain:

✔ Give your baby a cold object to chew and suck on (such as a washcloth, teething ring, or spoon).

✔ Use a homeopathic remedy like Hyland's teething tablets or gel. Hyland's teething remedies are 100 percent natural and safe to use (see www.earthbaby.com/hylands).

Illness is a sign that something is wrong and your body is trying to heal itself. Homeopathic remedies stimulate your body to heal itself.

Alleviating Chest and Sinus Congestion

While babies' immune systems are developing, they are especially vulnerable to catching colds. Common symptoms of colds include chest and sinus congestion. The goal in using massage to help congestion is to move the mucus out of the chest or sinus area, which enables your baby to feel and breathe better.

Knowing the difference: Cold versus flu

When your baby isn't feeling well, you may struggle to figure out whether she has a cold or the flu. We strongly recommend that you have your healthcare provider make a definitive diagnosis, but we also think it is important to understand the differences between the two because they have symptoms in common.

Colds

A cold is caused by one of more than 200 viruses (not bacteria). Most of the symptoms of a cold are above the neck. The most common symptoms are nasal stuffiness, a runny nose, and sneezing. Young babies and toddlers may carry a low-grade fever. Antibiotics are not used in treating colds; they may actually make the cold worse by killing helpful bacteria in the body.

Flu

The flu is caused by a single virus: the influenza. The symptoms of flu are all over the body, such as fever, body aches, lack of energy, and dizziness. In most cases, after a few days the body symptoms disappear, and the flu settles in the respiratory system with a hacking cough. Symptoms that resemble a cold usually emerge after the respiratory system becomes affected.

Massaging to ease chest congestion

To help alleviate chest congestion, keep your massage strokes moving toward your baby's head to push out any mucus that may be in the lungs.

You can use any of the chest-opening techniques that we show in Chapter 5:

- ✔ The Heart Stroke
- ✔ The Open Book Stroke
- ✔ The Butterfly Stroke

You can also use strokes on your baby's back, such as this one:

1. **Beginning from your baby's sacrum, using a Raking stroke (see Chapter 7) up toward your baby's head.** Your baby may either be lying down or sitting up and facing away from you.

2. **Add a tapping motion by using two fingers from one or both hands and tapping up your baby's back.**

   Your baby may begin to cough during these strokes. Coughing may be an indication that the massage is loosening up the mucus.

3. Place your baby on his back and open his arms up and out over his head to further open his chest and aid in breathing.

Massaging to ease sinus congestion

All the techniques in Chapter 6, which focuses on the face and neck, are useful in helping to drain the sinuses. You can also use the Sinus Relief Stroke:

1. Have your baby lying on his back or sitting up facing you.

2. Place two fingers from each hand on either side of the bridge of your baby's nose.

3. Sweep your fingers down and out under your baby's cheek bones, to pull out and down any mucus in the sinus.

Have tissues or a rubber bulb syringe handy when using this technique.

To further help your baby's breathing, use a drop or two of eucalyptus or peppermint essential oil in a vaporizer or your baby's bath.

Minimizing your baby's risk

You won't be able to prevent your baby from catching colds, but you can minimize her vulnerability to getting sick by practicing the following tips:

✔ Breastfeed your baby. Breastfed babies are sick less often than formula-fed babies because breast milk contains immune-building antibodies.

To ensure that your baby receives all the benefits of breast-feeding, the World Health Organization recommends breast-feeding for at least two years, and the American Academy of Pediatrics recommends breastfeeding for one year.

✔ If you have a newborn, make sure that you (and your friends and relatives) wash your hands often.

✔ Don't smoke around your baby.

✔ Keep your baby well hydrated.

Helping Your Fussy Baby

All babies are fussy from time to time, but some babies seem to be fussy more often than others. These babies don't have colic, and they also don't have any medical concerns. They're just. . .fussy!

Identifying fussy factors

Here are just some of the culprits that can make your baby fussy:

- ✔ Overstimulation
- ✔ Understimulation
- ✔ Hunger
- ✔ Tiredness
- ✔ Loneliness
- ✔ Being too hot
- ✔ Being too cold
- ✔ Diaper rash
- ✔ Food allergies
- ✔ Thrush
- ✔ Wet/soiled diaper
- ✔ Gastroesophageal reflux disease (GERD)

We could go on and on with this list, but we're sure you get the point: Your baby could be fussing over a lot of different things.

One important reason your baby may fuss is that she may not be getting her needs met. If you have a baby who needs to be held a lot, and she is kept in a mechanical swing or car seat for most of the day, you are going to have a fussy and unhappy baby.

Keep in mind that your baby is fussing in order to tell you something. You may not understand what she is telling you, so she gets more frustrated as she is trying to get her needs met and whatever you offer her is not what she is asking for.

Offering comfort through touch and massage

Fussy behavior can often be progressive. If you respond to your baby's requests early, you may manage to avoid your baby becoming upset. But if your baby has been telling you for a while that she needs something, and you haven't responded until the fussy behavior intensifies, you will have an upset baby to calm down.

Keep a log of your baby's fussy times. If you find that she fusses during a particular time of the day, plan ahead to give her a relaxing massage during that time. Relaxing her ahead of time may make her forget to be fussy.

Chances are that if you have been massaging your baby on a fairly regular basis, you are attuned to her needs and will respond to her requests promptly (before they become high pitched demands!). However, all babies (and adults, for that matter) do have fussy moments from time to time. Here we list ways to use touch and massage to calm and soothe your fussy baby:

- ✔ Wear your baby in a sling (see Chapter 1).

- ✔ Nurse in motion — nurse your baby while she is in a sling and you are on the go.

- ✔ Nurse frequently.

- ✔ Sing to your baby while you rock and gently dance with her.

- ✔ Carry your baby in the football hold (which we describe in the section "Massaging to ease colic" earlier in the chapter).

- ✔ Hold your baby over your shoulder and, with your free hand, make Raking strokes down his back (see Chapter 7).

- ✔ Place your baby sitting up on your lap, facing out. Push her forward a little (while your support her with one hand), and with your free hand make small circles down her back in a clockwise motion.

- ✔ Take a warm bath with your baby, followed by one of the after-bath massages we describe in Chapter 10.

Alternate ways to soothe your baby, just as you would if your baby had colic.

Avoid massaging your baby's face during a fussy episode. Face and head massages can overstimulate babies and may make them fussier.

Dealing with high need babies

High need babies are wired differently than other babies; they seem to be worried, intense, and easily overstimulated from birth. If you have a high need baby, in this section we show you ways to love your baby and take care of yourself.

Recognizing high need characteristics

Some parents think they have a baby with high needs until they meet other parents who really do! Here are some common characteristics that set high need babies apart from other babies:

- ✔ They are intense.
- ✔ They have high energy levels.
- ✔ They nurse frequently, sometimes several times an hour.
- ✔ They need to be held and comforted a lot.
- ✔ They are highly sensitive.
- ✔ They awaken frequently.
- ✔ They are demanding.
- ✔ They refuse to be left alone in a car seat, swing, or bouncer.

Loving a high need baby

If you have figured out that yours truly is a high need baby, you need a change of perspective: Try to consider yourself blessed to have such a special baby! The situation doesn't have to be negative. These babies are definitely challenging, but they are easy to love if you let go of expectations you may have about how your baby "should" be. Your relationship with your high need baby can bring out the best in both of you.

Here are some ways you can love your high need baby:

- ✔ **Listen to him.** High need babies don't give up until their needs are met. So if your baby doesn't stop crying unless you are holding him all the time, invest in a sling and carry him around with you.
- ✔ **Share sleep with your baby.** Co-sleeping (see Chapter 3) makes it easier for you to keep up with all the extra feedings and night wakening, while making it possible for you to get the sleep you need.
- ✔ **Bathe with your baby.** See Chapter 10 for tips on doing so safely.

> ✔ **Massage your baby!** High need babies usually thrive on a lot of touch, so use your massage skills frequently.

Following is a massage sequence — the High Contact Massage — that your high need baby will be sure to love. Your baby is on his back and able to see you throughout the entire sequence, which is filled with gliding, gentle strokes to help soothe your little one.

Be sure to talk lovingly to your baby during this massage. He will be delighted by all you are able to give him.

> ✔ The Dolphin Stroke (see Chapter 4)
>
> ✔ The Taffy Pull (see Chapter 5)
>
> ✔ Ankles Away (see Chapter 5)
>
> ✔ This Little Piggy (see Chapter 5)
>
> ✔ I Love You (see Chapter 5)
>
> ✔ The Heart Stroke (see Chapter 5)
>
> ✔ The Open Book Stroke on the chest (see Chapter 5)
>
> ✔ Alternating Hands (see Chapter 5)
>
> ✔ Hand stroking (see Chapter 5)
>
> ✔ Finger stroking (see Chapter 5)
>
> ✔ Circling the Eyes (see Chapter 6)
>
> ✔ The Open Book Stroke on the forehead (see Chapter 6)

Be sure to finish with lots of cuddling. Keep in mind that this sequence contains a lot of techniques: Trust your instincts, and skip any strokes that don't feel right to you or your baby.

Comforting yourself

Much like having a baby with colic, having a high need baby can take a toll on you and your family over time. Don't forget to take steps to lower your own stress level whenever you feel yourself getting frustrated:

> ✔ Ask for help when you need it.
>
> ✔ Take care of your own physical and emotional needs.
>
> ✔ Find some alone time — time when you are not taking care of anyone but yourself.

Healing Your Baby's Skin

Babies are prone to dry skin because their oil-producing glands aren't fully developed yet. Frequent bathing, dry air, static electricity, and harsh detergents can also contribute to dry skin.

If your baby has dry skin, you can use massage as an opportunity to rehydrate your baby's skin. Here's how:

- ✔ Massage your baby after bathing. Be sure to keep your bath time short; the hot water could be drying out your baby's skin.

- ✔ Use only 100 percent natural oils (see Chapter 4), which will not affect your baby's sensitive skin.

- ✔ If your baby's skin is very dry, consider massaging him with oil twice a day. Even if you are short on time, you can do this by incorporating massage on the changing table (see Chapter 10).

Following are a few additional ways to protect your baby's skin:

- ✔ Use only gentle baby soaps and shampoos on your baby's skin. You may also want to switch to a mild laundry detergent.

- ✔ Run a humidifier during the winter months. The extra moisture will not only help your baby's skin but may also prevent her from catching a cold.

- ✔ Nurse your baby frequently. If you are formula-feeding your baby, you may need to give her a daily water bottle.

- ✔ If you are a breastfeeding mother, try increasing the Omega 3 fatty acids in your diet, which are found in salmon, flax seed oil, canola oil, or supplements.

Treating eczema

Eczema is one of the most common forms of rashes that children have. It is a form of dermatitis caused by a combination of genetic and environmental factors. An overreactive immune system responds to certain environmental or food allergies with very dry skin and a rash.

Some symptoms of eczema are:

- ✔ Tiny white bumps that you can feel on the skin

- ✔ Dry white or red patches on the skin

- ✔ Frequent flare-ups when the dry skin patches and bumps may become irritated and oozy

If your baby has eczema, talk with your pediatrician about treatment options. Here are some suggestions for caring for his skin:

✔ Bathe your baby in short, lukewarm (not hot) baths. Avoid using soap unless you absolutely need to. During an eczema flare-up, your baby may not be able to tolerate a bath at all. In this situation, use a water-free cleanser.

✔ After a bath, pat your baby dry with a very soft towel — 100 percent cotton is best. Never rub excessively.

✔ Always follow a bath with a massage using a heavy (and gentle) moisturizing cream or lotion, such as Kiehl's Baby Nurturing Cream for Face and Body (see www.kiehls.com) or Little Forest Natural Products for Baby Skin Care (see www.littleforest.com). Massage the cream into your baby's damp skin.

✔ Use a humidifier.

✔ Use only 100 percent cotton clothing and sheets for your baby. Especially avoid wool.

✔ Breastfeed your baby if possible, and delay introducing solids until he is at least 6 months old.

Caring for cradle cap

Cradle cap is a rash found on the scalps of many babies beginning between birth and 3 months. The skin cells of newborns can grow faster than they fall off, leaving a crusty layer.

Seborrhea is a skin condition that can show up behind the ears or on the knees, underarms, eyelids, face, neck, or diaper area. When it occurs on top of the head, it is called *cradle cap*. Forms of seborrhea on teenagers and adults can include dandruff and dry flaking skin.

You can use a gentle scalp massage along with oil to treat cradle cap. Here's how:

1. **Use a mild oil, such as vegetable or olive oil, for most cases of cradle cap. Heavier oils may leave a residue that could irritate the cradle cap.**

2. **Massage the oil onto your baby's scalp using gentle but vigorous strokes.**

3. **Leave the oil on your baby's scalp for about 10 to 15 minutes.** You can use this time to massage the rest of your baby's body.

4. **Use a soft toothbrush or baby's hair brush to gently loosen the skin.**

5. **Wash your baby's hair with a mild baby shampoo.**

Use this treatment on your baby a couple times each week until the cradle cap disappears. Be sure to massage gently over your baby's soft spot.

Most cases of cradle cap disappear by the time the baby turns 1.

Chapter 12

Massage for Emotional and Developmental Issues

In This Chapter
▶ Aiding attachment with massage
▶ Handling developmental delays
▶ Managing sibling relationships

*I*f you've read some or all of the chapters that come before this, you are already aware that infant massage has many benefits. (If you haven't read it, Chapter 2 offers a great introduction to this topic.) In this chapter, we take you deeper into a discussion of the benefits of massage — specifically the emotional benefits.

In this chapter, we discuss what attachment really means in a baby's world, how circumstances such as adoption and foster parenting affect attachment, and how to strengthen your relationship with your baby. We also show you that massage is an important tool in a parenting style that emphasizes bonding and interdependence. Finally, we explore how to use massage to help a developmentally delayed baby in concrete ways.

Overcoming Attachment Issues

When you bond with your baby, you are creating a relationship based on love and trust. That bond is tested throughout your baby's development, but if your attachment with your baby is strong, the bond will only grow with time.

In Chapter 1, we talk about using an *attachment parenting* style. Attachment is created by showing your baby affection, mirroring and reflecting your baby's emotions, touching him, helping him soothe himself during times of stress, and nurturing him. Attachment is a process that both you and your baby participate in, and the quality of the attachment is determined by how sensitive you are and how responsive your baby is.

We offer suggestions throughout this book for ways to use massage and other techniques to build attachment with your baby. But in some circumstances, building attachment is especially challenging. For example, babies and older children who have been placed for adoption or who are in foster care have unique needs. Because they have already experienced profound loss and separation, creating a foundation of trust in order to develop an attachment can be difficult.

In the sections that follow, we show you how to use massage and touch to help create trust in order to form attachments even in these challenging situations.

Recognizing patterns of attachment

Not surprisingly, research shows that parenting styles affect the quality of attachment between parents and their children. Adopted and foster children may come to their new parents with an existing pattern of attachment — meaning that their ability to bond has already been influenced by the parent(s) they knew before you.

We want you to be familiar with patterns of attachment so you can not only recognize them but redirect them in healthy ways using touch and massage.

The way that a baby or child attaches to a caregiver forms the basis of her relationships throughout her adult life. We don't say this to create stress for you — only to emphasize how crucial it is that you take every step possible to create a positive attachment with your little one. (As you prepare to be the best parent or caregiver possible, we strongly encourage you to reflect on your own childhood and how it may influence your parenting style.)

Securely attached babies

Sensitive caregivers generally produce securely attached babies. What does it mean to be a sensitive caregiver?

- ✔ Having the ability to see things from the baby's perspective
- ✔ Responding to the baby's needs promptly
- ✔ Being consistent and positive

> ✔ Tending to leave a contented baby alone during play, and
>   responding supportively when the baby needs help with diffi-
>   cult emotions, such as frustration or anger

Securely attached babies look to their caregivers for comfort.
When they're upset, if their caregivers are nearby they are usually
easily calmed down.

Insecurely attached babies

Insensitive caregivers often create insecure attachments with their
babies. What are the characteristics of insensitive caregivers?

> ✔ They respond to their babies' needs based on the caregivers'
>   feelings and needs.
>
> ✔ They are inconsistent.
>
> ✔ They reinforce positive behaviors and ignore negative ones.
>   In a misguided effort to teach children how to control their
>   behavior, insensitive parents teach their children rejection.

Insecurely attached babies may ignore, actively resist, or cling to
their caregivers.

Bonding with an adopted or foster child

Even if you are a sensitive parent, your adopted or foster baby may
come to you with an insecure attachment pattern. Or perhaps after
reading the previous section you recognize that you exhibit some
characteristics of an insensitive caregiver. Either way, you can
work to improve your situation by recognizing these attachment
patterns and taking action to bond with your new addition in a
positive way.

Attachment is co-created: The combination of your child's temperament and your sensitivity determines the quality of attachment.

Adopting a newborn or infant

So if you've adopted a newborn or infant, where do you begin the
bonding process? Cuddling, holding, massaging, touching, stroking,
kissing, and hugging are all wonderful ways to create an attachment.
The more often you touch your baby in a nurturing way, the sooner
you will build the trusting relationship you need to form a secure
attachment.

Here are some suggestions:

- ✔ Wear your baby in a sling (see Chapter 1).
- ✔ Avoid separations if possible.
- ✔ Make a lot of eye contact.
- ✔ Co-sleep (see Chapter 3).
- ✔ Massage your baby every chance you get:
  - • Before and/or after baths
  - • On the changing table
  - • Before naps
  - • While she is in the sling
  - • During breaks from long drives in the car
- ✔ Nurse your baby often.

  Does this seem like strange advice? Yes, it is possible for some women to breastfeed an adopted baby. If you're interested in finding out how, visit the La Leche League Web site (www.lalecheleague.org) for more information, or see *Breastfeeding For Dummies* by Sharon Perkins and Carol Vannais (Wiley).

- ✔ Bathe with your baby (see Chapter 10).

- ✔ Give your baby a *transferential object* — a fancy name for a blanket or stuffed animal that he can hold during times when you can't hold him.

  Sleep with the transferential object before giving it to your baby so the object picks up your smell.

Adopting an older baby or child

Older babies and children obviously bring more experiences and history with them than babies do. Some of these experiences may include trauma, abuse, and neglect. Children with this type of background need you to show them how to bond and attach. You can respectfully and sensitively bring safe touch and massage to the relationship.

Here are some suggestions to get you started:

- ✔ Avoid separations until you have a secure attachment with your child.

- ✔ Go slowly. Don't overwhelm your child with a lot of touch. Respect her boundaries and her right to say no, but don't stop trying to touch your child.

✔ Include siblings and other family members in creating safe and appropriate touch (see Chapter 9).

✔ Massage your older baby's feet. The feet are often a safe and noninvasive place to start massaging your child.

✔ Co-sleep if you can. If doing so creates too much closeness for your child, read to her before sleep, and stay in bed with her until she falls asleep. Or simply try watching television with your older child while you are both lying in bed.

✔ Make a lot of eye contact.

✔ Respond to tantrums appropriately; don't ignore the behavior (see Chapter 9).

✔ Rock your child in a rocking chair.

✔ Comb or brush her hair.

✔ Go swimming together.

✔ Dance!

Adopting a child from another country

In the United States, international adoption has become very popular. In 2002, approximately 20,000 international children were adopted by U.S. citizens.

International adoption allows you the opportunity to love and parent a child who desperately needs a home and family. But when you adopt a child from another country, attachment may bring special challenges. Here are some obstacles you want to prepare for:

✔ You and your child may speak different languages.

✔ You may learn little or nothing about your child's background and medical history.

✔ If your child has been institutionalized prior to adoption, he may be developmentally delayed.

✔ If you adopt an older baby or child, the transition into your home will seem sudden. Cognitively, your child may not be developed enough to understand why she is living in a new home.

✔ Everything your child experiences after coming to live with you will be new: He'll need to adjust to a new country, culture, language, food, and smells.

Children who live in institutions in other countries are often used to very rigid routines, little or no emotional and sensory contact, and neglect. (In some Eastern European countries, orphanages have only one caretaker per 50 infants.) Most of these babies live in institutions because their parents are extremely poor; their families literally cannot afford to feed them. Living in an orphanage for even a short period of time may profoundly affect a baby's or child's ability to attach.

Do not lose hope. Many children who have lived in institutions do very well after being placed with a loving family. It takes time to deinstitutionalize your child. He needs a lot of physical and emotional contact with you to be able to reattach.

Here are some ways you can make your child's transition easier:

- ✔ Have a cuddly transitional object (a blanket or stuffed animal) ready for your child right away.

- ✔ Plan on sleeping in the same room as your child at first; he's probably used to sleeping with a roomful of other children.

- ✔ Realize that you are responsible for teaching your baby about touch: when, where, and how.

- ✔ Find out about your baby's cultural attitudes regarding touch before you bring him home.

- ✔ Be careful not to overstimulate your new baby.

- ✔ Avoid separations.

- ✔ Recognize that your baby may reject your touch at first due to sensory defensiveness. Don't take it personally or give up.

- ✔ Create and stick to a routine.

- ✔ Use play with objects that have different textures and shapes to introduce touch and provide an opportunity for physical closeness.

- ✔ Plan on you and your partner being your child's only caretakers at first.

Caring for a foster child

More than 500,000 children are in foster care in the United States, and only about half will be returned to their families. Some babies and children in foster care have been placed for adoption and are waiting for a family. Others have been removed from their biological families because they have been abused or neglected or their parents have died.

When you become a foster parent, you must keep two critical issues in mind:

✔ Unless you plan to adopt, the child's placement with you is temporary.

✔ The child may have an attachment related disorder when she is placed with you.

Even though your foster child may be moving on to a permanent home soon, it is important for you to use touch in your relationship. You want to begin with safe, noninvasive touch, especially if your foster child has experienced trauma or abuse. Even newborns can be hypersensitive to touch and may find even a little contact too much too soon.

Many of the suggestions we offer in the previous sections on bonding with adopted babies also work with foster children. Keep in mind that to create a trusting relationship you must respect the child's boundaries, but don't give up if he rejects physical contact at first.

Children who have loving and sensitive foster parents are more likely to flourish in permanent homes.

Dealing with Reactive Attachment Disorder

Children diagnosed with Reactive Attachment Disorder (RAD) have experienced extreme chaos, neglect, deprivation, and abuse in their early lives. They may become violent, fearful, and hypervigilant.

Symptoms of RAD, which can be seen even in babies, include the following:

✔ Constant crying or colic

✔ Failure to thrive

✔ Refusal to be comforted or held

✔ Little to no responsiveness; the baby does not even return smiles

✔ A tendency to become enraged when held

✔ A preference for being left alone in a playpen rather than being held

Babies and children with RAD physiologically cannot calm themselves down. They are in a constant state of terror and react violently to their feelings.

If you suspect that your adopted or foster baby has RAD, you need to seek professional help. Treating an attachment disorder typically requires working with a team of professionals. You can find more information about RAD and where to find appropriate treatment at the Institute for Attachment & Child Development's Web site: www.instituteforattachment.org.

Ultimately, direct approaches using safe and nurturing touch, along with physical and emotional contact, will help your baby heal from trauma.

Coping with Developmental Delays

When babies lag behind in expected developmental milestones (such as those we discuss in Chapter 3), they may be considered developmentally delayed. Babies and children may experience delays in all areas or in specific areas. Some babies catch up to their expected abilities, while others have limitations for their whole lives. Whether a delay becomes a disability may depend on whether the baby receives needed resources or on the cause and seriousness of the delay.

Delays can affect your baby's gross and fine motor skills, speech, language, and social skills. Global delays occur when all areas of development are affected.

Identifying causes of developmental delays

Some frequent causes of developmental delays include:

- Premature birth
- Low birth weight
- Down syndrome
- Fetal alcohol syndrome
- Mental retardation
- Neglect and physical abuse

> ✔ Cerebral palsy
> ✔ Rett syndrome

Realizing effects on attachment

As we explain earlier in this chapter, attachment is a reciprocal dance between parents and their baby. Developmental delays can affect your ability to attach and bond with your baby.

It is challenging to form an attachment with a baby who is unable to return a smile or coo, or a baby who can't hear you speak lovingly to him. Part of the dance of attachment involves responding to your baby responding to you. Babies with developmental delays may not be able to respond in ways you expect, if at all. All babies need to form secure attachments, but babies with delays need you to work even harder.

When you have a baby who experiences developmental delays, touch may be your most important tool of communication.

Trusting the benefits of touch and massage

Because developmentally delayed babies may have both health issues and attachment concerns, you may need to address both. (See Chapter 11 for information about using massage to address health issues.)

Massage can help you accomplish the following:

> ✔ Lower your baby's stress levels
> ✔ Communicate with your baby
> ✔ Create a bond and attachment
> ✔ Learn to accept your baby's limitations and appreciate new gains in development
> ✔ Discover what your baby needs
> ✔ Stimulate learning
> ✔ Encourage your baby to gain weight
> ✔ Feel less helpless
> ✔ Strengthen your baby's immune system

Some developmental delays specifically affect muscle tone. As we explain in the following section, you can use massage to either stimulate or relax muscle tone, depending on your baby's condition.

Working with muscle tone

Muscle tone is what allows us to move. Muscles may be either soft or tense. Some developmentally delayed babies have very loose or floppy muscle tone, while others have stiff, tense muscles.

Hypotonia refers to muscles that are loose and limp. *Hypertonia* refers to overly tense and tightened muscles. Some babies alternate between loose and limp muscles and very tense muscles.

Premature babies may experience hypertonia or hypotonia, as well as babies with the following conditions:

- ✔ Cerebral palsy
- ✔ Fetal alcohol syndrome
- ✔ Down syndrome
- ✔ Mental retardation

We discuss massaging premature infants in Chapter 8, and we cover fetal alcohol syndrome in Chapter 13. Here, we focus on using massage for babies with Down syndrome, cerebral palsy, and mental retardation.

Down syndrome

Down syndrome is the most frequently diagnosed cause for developmental delays. Approximately 5,000 babies born in the United States each year have Down syndrome. According to the National Down Syndrome Society, 80 percent of babies born with Down syndrome are born to women younger than age 25. That's because the majority of births occur with women in this age group. The risk of Down syndrome actually increases with a woman's age; the incidence of Down syndrome rises dramatically for women over 35.

Causes and prevention

Down syndrome is caused by a chromosomal abnormality. Although different types of Down syndrome exist, all involve an error in cell division. The most common type of Down syndrome involves a baby being born with three copies of chromosome 21.

Research indicates that some cases of Down syndrome may be due to inadequate supplies of *folic acid,* a B vitamin. Mothers who have a low supply of folic acid have a 300 percent higher chance of having a baby with Down syndrome.

Folic acid helps to support the rapid growth of cells during pregnancy. Your amino acids need folic acid to aid in conversion. Without it, you end up with too much *homocysteine* in your blood, which is thought to create birth defects. Your baby needs folic acid for the proper functioning and production of DNA.

Start taking 400 mcg of folic acid a day before you plan on conceiving. After you get pregnant, take 600 to 800 mcg of folic acid a day. (Most prenatal vitamins contain 1,000 mcg.)

Here are some common food sources of folic acid:

✓ Dark, leafy green vegetables, including broccoli, asparagus, and collard greens

✓ Lentils and chickpeas

✓ Oranges, bananas, and strawberries

✓ Carrots, tomatoes, and potatoes

✓ Fortified grains and cereals

✓ Nuts

✓ Eggs and milk

✓ Fish

Symptoms

Down syndrome can cause many different symptoms. Some newborns have only a few; others have many. Here are a few common physical expressions of Down syndrome:

✓ Loose, limp muscles (muscle hypotonia)

✓ Eyes that slant upward

✓ Hyperflexibility

✓ Abnormally shaped ears

✓ A flat area on the back of the head

If your doctor suspects that your newborn has Down syndrome, she will most likely order a *karotype,* an analysis of the baby's chromosomes, to confirm the diagnosis.

Some of the major medical problems associated with Down syndrome are:

- Heart defects
- Weakened immunity
- Hearing and vision problems
- Intellectual handicaps
- Digestive problems
- Proneness to spinal injuries due to weakened vertebrae

Massage techniques to use

If your baby has Down syndrome, consult with your pediatrician to find out if there are any strokes you may need to avoid using, especially if your baby has a heart problem.

A key thing to keep in mind is to use gentle massage techniques on a baby with Down syndrome. The following techniques are appropriate:

- The Dolphin Stroke (see Chapter 4)
- The Ear Stroke (see Chapter 6)
- The Taffy Pull (see Chapters 5 and 7)
- Ankles Away (see Chapters 5 and 7)
- This Little Piggy (see Chapter 5)
- Raking (see Chapters 5 and 7)
- Sun and Moon (see Chapter 5)
- I Love You (see Chapter 5)
- The Open Book Stroke (see Chapters 5 and 6)
- Alternating Hands (see Chapter 5)
- Thumb Circles (see Chapter 5)
- Hands stroking (see Chapter 5)
- Finger stroking (see Chapter 5)

Go slowly, and introduce techniques one or two at a time. Just a minute or two of massage, followed by holding and cuddling, may be enough with a developmentally delayed newborn.

Here are some more tips to keep in mind with your Down syndrome baby:

 ✔ Dry skin is a problem for babies with Down syndrome. You can find tips on how to handle dry skin in Chapter 11.

 ✔ Babies with Down syndrome have difficulty regulating their body temperature. You can massage your baby with his clothes on, but make sure he doesn't overheat.

 ✔ Down syndrome creates sinus and chest infections. See Chapter 11 for tips on dealing with these ailments, and consider running a humidifier in your baby's room.

 ✔ Frequent massage helps your baby develop muscle tone.

Cerebral palsy

Cerebral palsy (CP) is caused by brain injury or abnormal brain development that occurs either before birth or within the first two to three years of life. The United Cerebral Palsy Association estimates that 500,000 people in the United States have CP.

Causes

CP is caused by an injury to the part of the brain that controls movement. Following are some common causes of this type of injury:

 ✔ Severe oxygen shortage to the brain

 ✔ Jaundice

 ✔ Rh incompatibility

 ✔ Infections during pregnancy

Babies with CP are unable to control their movements and posture. Some babies with CP may have learning problems, mental retardation, or difficulty seeing. CP is not a progressive disorder.

Types of CP

There are three types of CP:

 ✔ **Spastic:** The muscles are very tight and movement is stiff, especially in the legs. Babies with spastic CP cannot relax their muscles.

 ✔ **Athetoid:** Movement throughout the entire body is affected. Movement is slow and uncontrolled with low muscle tone.

✔ **Mixed:** Involves both too much and too little muscle tone. Movement is stiff and difficult to control, making balance and coordination difficult to impossible.

Babies and children with CP are at risk for seizures. Seizures are a sign that the nervous system is not working correctly. Seizures can be difficult to notice in a newborn or baby. Here are some signs that your baby may be having a seizure:

✔ His eyes are rolling.

✔ His body is stiff.

✔ He is crying in a way that sounds very different than usual.

✔ His arms and legs are moving in a jerking fashion.

✔ He is staring.

✔ His movements look unnatural.

✔ His skin color changes.

✔ He stops breathing.

If your baby has a seizure, here's what you need to do:

✔ Try to stay calm and breathe.

✔ Turn your baby onto his side.

✔ Make sure there is nothing in his mouth.

✔ Place your hand on him for comfort, but don't try to stop the jerking.

✔ After the seizure is over, hold and cuddle your baby while you call the doctor.

Seizures aren't necessarily dangerous, but they are very scary to watch.

Treatment

Babies develop remarkably fast during their first few years. If your baby has CP, it is important to receive intervention as soon as possible. Seeking intervention can make a dramatic difference in your baby's development.

There isn't a cure for CP, but treatment for children can help reduce the effects of the brain injury. Physical and speech therapy, along with equipment such as braces and splints, are helpful. Ask your doctor to show you how to do physical therapy exercises with your newborn at home.

Some parents find that acupuncture and CranioSacral Therapy are effective treatments for the symptoms of CP. Acupuncture balances and stimulates the flow of energy *(Oi)* throughout the body's *meridians,* or energy channels. Acupuncturists either use fine, sterile needles to stimulate energy flow at acupuncture points (the specific places where the meridians are easily located), apply heat to these points, or use a technique called *cupping.* Cupping stimulates points through suction, with the use of a jar. To find an acupuncturist in your area, log onto www.acupuncture.com.

CranioSacral Therapy is a gentle and powerful hands-on therapy that improves central nervous system functioning and reduces stress. The gentle touch helps to balance the cerebrospinal fluid and the tissues around the brain and spinal cord. You can learn more about CranioSacral Therapy or find a therapist in your area at The Upledger Institute's Web site: www.upledger.com.

Massage and touch techniques to use

Massaging your baby with CP can help to reduce muscle tone, increase muscle control, and improve posture. Regular massage therapy with your baby can also improve brain and body communication.

Here are some techniques you can use on your baby with CP:

- ✔ Help your baby's posture by teaching her how to sit. In Chapter 14, we show you how.

- ✔ Stretch your baby's arms and legs to prevent *contractures* (shortening of the muscles). You can find these stretches in Chapter 14.

- ✔ Avoid constipation, a common effect of CP, by using the techniques we discuss in Chapter 11.

- ✔ Use any of the massage techniques we show in this book to alleviate pain from muscle contractions.

Your baby may be hypersensitive to both touch and stimuli. Be sure to move slowly and gently and watch her cues.

Mental retardation

People who are mentally retarded have a below-normal IQ (less than 75) and have considerable difficulty functioning in everyday life. Statistics show that 3 out of 100 people have some level of mental retardation (MR). MR is 10 times more common than cerebral palsy.

The severity of someone's MR used to be determined solely by an IQ score. Today, the severity of the MR is determined by how much assistance a person needs. People with MR may need intermittent, limited, extensive, or pervasive support.

The majority of people with MR have only a mild level of retardation. They are a little slower than the average person, but most people wouldn't even notice that they have MR.

Causes and prevention

A few factors may cause mental retardation, including:

- ✔ Genetics
- ✔ Severe malnutrition
- ✔ Maternal health problems
- ✔ Health problems with the baby
- ✔ A difficult birth

Fetal alcohol syndrome (FAS) is a common cause of MR in babies. We cover FAS in Chapter 13.

Many screening tests are available that, if performed early, may detect a health issue that could progress into MR. Ask your doctor about these tests.

Symptoms

Because there are many different reasons your baby may have MR, it may be difficult to diagnose a newborn. Some of the symptoms won't present themselves until your baby reaches school age and her level of intelligence and ability becomes more obvious.

Common signs that something could be wrong are the same as signs that your baby is developmentally delayed:

- ✔ Your baby sits, crawls, or walks far behind schedule.
- ✔ She has a very difficult time learning to speak.
- ✔ She has difficulty feeding.

Some toddlers with mental retardation or autism bang their heads against something before they go to bed, usually in an effort to self-soothe. If your toddler is into head-banging, there are some ways you can help her:

✔ Create a relaxing bedtime routine by combining massage with a warm bath to teach her how to self-soothe.

✔ Sometimes babies who bang their heads love rhythm. Find music that your baby enjoys. Play it and dance with your baby before bath, massage, and bedtime.

Tools for parenting a baby with MR

Your baby with MR needs extra love and attention from you. Children with MR are at a high risk for low self-esteem as they grow. They can tell that they are different from other children and won't have the same life that others do.

Children with MR also need extra help learning the following:

✔ How to take care of themselves (such as dressing, feeding, and going to the bathroom)

✔ How to communicate

✔ How to respect boundaries

✔ How to interact socially (including how to play)

Can babies learn sign language?

The answer is *absolutely*. Teaching babies sign language gives them an important communication tool to use before they are able to speak. Have you seen a 10-month-old wave goodbye? Babies learn to wave through repetition. Every time you or a family member leaves, you wave and say "bye bye." Pretty soon, your baby starts to wave back.

You can begin teaching your baby to sign at any age, and you can expect to see results when they are between 7 and 9 months old. You don't have to know American Sign Language either. You can simply make up simple hand gestures as a form of communication.

Why sign with your baby? Here are some advantages:

✔ Your baby will be less frustrated as he is able to communicate his needs easily.

✔ Signing stimulates learning.

✔ Signing can be fun.

✔ It enhances your bonding and relationship.

If you would like to find out more about how to teach your baby sign language, log onto www.signingbaby.com or www.babysigns.com.

Most people with MR can lead productive and fulfilling lives. You can assure a fulfilling life for your baby by providing him with all the love and support he needs. Here are some ideas for accomplishing this goal:

- Practice attachment parenting (see Chapter 1).

- Encourage your toddler's independence.

- Hold, cuddle, and touch your baby as much as you can.

- Use massage to teach your older baby about boundaries and touch.

- Have realistic expectations.

- Teach your baby sign language (see the sidebar "Can babies learn sign language?").

Handling Special Needs and Siblings

Jealousy is normal when a child learns that another baby is on the way. And when you bring a special needs baby into your home, the jealousy can intensify. If your new baby has a disability, it can have a profound effect on your family. Plus, your other children may not understand what is wrong with the new baby.

Being honest

It's important for you to communicate honestly with your children about the new baby. Use words they will understand, and keep things simple.

Tell your children the truth, and encourage them to express their feelings. Being honest with your children helps them to feel like equal members of the family. It's your job to help your children cope with what they are feeling.

For example, if you have an older birth child and are adopting a baby, you need to explain what adoption is. You can start by saying, "Adoption is when a baby lives with another family after being born." As your children grow older, plan on adding more of the truth to the statement: "Your brother's birth mother wasn't able to take care of him, and that's why we adopted him."

If your new child has a disability, you need to explain to your other children everything you can about the condition: What it will be like for the child, how her health may affect the family, and how any changes that may need to be made will affect your other children.

Minimizing rivalry

Even though your new baby has special needs and may require a lot of attention and outside support, make sure that you don't give your new baby all your attention. Even though this baby has special needs, he doesn't need to be your favorite. If you are giving him all your attention, he will grow to feel like the favorite, and your other children will feel that way, too. You will be setting the stage for resentments, competition, and conflicts between your children.

Here are some ways you can minimize sibling rivalry:

- ✔ Enlist the help of your child(ren) in preparing for your new baby's arrival. For example, if your new baby will have a nursery, ask your child(ren) to help decorate it.

- ✔ If you are adopting a baby from another culture, share learning about that culture with your child(ren).

- ✔ Teach your child(ren) how to give the new sibling a massage (see Chapter 9).

- ✔ Keep in mind that siblings can co-sleep, too! (See Chapter 3 for more on co-sleeping.)

- ✔ Understand that your new baby's disability is stressful on your other children.

If you have been giving your children massages and practicing other tools of attachment parenting, they are more likely to be compassionate and sensitive. In other words, your children are more likely to regard the presence of a new baby with special needs as a gift.

Don't worry about treating all your children exactly the same. Celebrate the differences between them by highlighting their special skills and uniqueness.

Chapter 13

Massage for High Risk Babies

•••

In This Chapter

▶ Helping babies addicted to drugs and alcohol

▶ Assisting babies affected by HIV and AIDS

▶ Using resources to help you and your baby

•••

The unfortunate truth is that poor prenatal judgment can and does expose babies to drugs, alcohol, and HIV. Too many newborns still suffer from the effects of their mothers' decisions to take drugs and consume alcohol and from exposure to the HIV virus in utero.

Babies born in these circumstances need a lot of extra attention and compassion. In this chapter, we show how touch and massage can help give these babies a fighting chance of survival.

Babies Born to Addiction

Unborn babies are vulnerable to the care their mothers give them. If a mother uses drugs or alcohol during pregnancy, chances are her baby will be born with a lot of problems. The good news is that massaging a drug- or alcohol-affected baby can have a strong positive impact on the health of the baby and on the parent–child relationship.

Helping the drug-addicted baby

Even over-the-counter drugs can affect the health of an unborn baby. For example, aspirin taken during the last trimester of pregnancy may increase the likelihood of a stillbirth or prolong labor.

And certain prescription drugs are addictive to a fetus and lead to withdrawal symptoms after birth; the number of babies being born addicted to oxycodone, for example, is increasing rapidly.

You can imagine, then, the dangerous impact of illegal substances on a baby's health.

Short- and long-term symptoms

Drug withdrawal is a serious and sometimes dangerous experience. A baby who is born drug-addicted craves the drug that her mother used. Because the drug is no longer available, the baby's central nervous system is overstimulated, producing withdrawal symptoms. Adults who are addicted to drugs often feel terrified of withdrawal. Imagine a baby born with the same feelings, only without the cognitive ability to understand where they came from.

Babies born with drug addictions may have the following symptoms:

✔ Uncontrollable shaking and sweating

✔ Vomiting

✔ Diarrhea

✔ Nonstop crying

✔ Difficulty nursing

✔ Seizures

✔ A smaller head size than is normal for a newborn

✔ An increased risk for sudden infant death syndrome (SIDS)

✔ Proneness to respiratory distress

✔ Strokes

After the immediate concerns of the drug withdrawal are taken care of, the addicted baby is still at risk for long-term effects. Some of these effects include:

✔ An inability to regulate emotions

✔ An inability to delay gratification

✔ Poor impulse control

✔ Social problems

✔ Difficulty focusing

Often the drug-addicted baby's mother may be going through withdrawal as well. If this happens, the newborn may be faced with the additional trauma of being placed in foster care. If he does stay in his mother's care, her ability to be emotionally available to her baby is diminished.

 So in addition to the physical effects of the drugs, these babies often suffer from separation or emotional abandonment from their mothers. The effects of an insecure attachment (which we discuss in Chapter 12) can last a lifetime.

Benefits of massage and touch

Many drug-addicted babies spend a good deal of time in the hospital, where they are treated for withdrawal. Much of the treatment they receive is the same as for a premature baby (see Chapter 8). The difference is that many of these babies may be given Valium, phenobarbital, or Thorazine to ease the suffering of the withdrawal.

 It may take up to a month for a drug-addicted baby to go through withdrawal. Any touch this baby receives will take place in a neonatal intensive care unit (NICU). These babies need to be treated very gently and carefully; they are fragile. Some drug-addicted babies go into spasms and convulsions just from being touched.

The effects of epidurals on newborns

You may not want to think of an epidural as a drug that affects your baby, but it is. An epidural is injected into the lumbar region of the mother's spine. A large amount of the drug enters her bloodstream and passes through the placenta, where it enters the baby's circulatory system. Although epidurals are widely used by many doctors and hospitals, the effects of the drug have not been adequately studied or routinely talked about. Epidurals can cause the following effects in newborns:

✔ Lack of responsiveness

✔ Decreased visual skills and alertness

✔ Breastfeeding difficulties

✔ Decreased heart rate

In addition, an epidural decreases the mother's ability to push, which raises the incidence of using forceps or vacuums during delivery.

Some studies have indicated a correlation between drugs used during labor and addiction problems for the baby later in life. Obviously, more research is necessary, but we strongly encourage you to ask lots of questions of your doctor and nurses before making the decision to use drugs during delivery.

The Hale House

"These babies don't know anything but fear and pain. I try and change that."
Mother Hale

The Hale House is a nonprofit organization that offers free supportive services to families in trouble in Harlem, New York. The Hale House began through the work of one woman, Clara McBride Hale, known simply as Mother Hale. In the late 1960s, while running a day and respite care program from her home, Mother Hale took in an infant whose mother was addicted to heroin.

Mother Hale created the Hale House Center for the Promotion of Human Development, Inc., in 1972, in part to offer help to babies who are either affected by drugs and alcohol or addicted to these substances.

Mother Hale passed away in 1992. The Hale House continues to run, led by her daughter, Dr. Lorraine Hale. Today it is flourishing under the care of a board of directors, Executive Director Randolph McLaughlin, Esq., and a dedicated staff.

Services at the Hale House have expanded over the years to include offering help and programs to children whose parents are incarcerated or infected with HIV or AIDS, and to babies and children who need loving homes.

If you'd like to learn more about the remarkable work of the Hale House, you can reach its staff at 212-663-0700 or visit www.HaleHouse.org.

When a drug-addicted baby is through withdrawal (and out of danger), you can begin to use some of the massage techniques we show in this book. Be sure to keep the following in mind during your massage:

✔ Keep the stimulation level low. Make sure the lights are dim, and avoid playing music. (You may be able to hum or sing softly during the massage.)

Watch closely for signs that your baby is overstimulated (see Chapter 4). You want to stop any activity before your baby becomes distressed.

✔ Use only gentle massage techniques. The following strokes are safe to use:

   • The Dolphin Stroke (see Chapter 4)

   • Ears to Chin (see Chapter 6)

   • Circling the Eyes (see Chapter 6)

   • The Open Book Stroke on the forehead (see Chapter 6)

   • The Ear Stroke (see Chapter 6)

- Chinny Chin Chin (see Chapter 6)
- Small Circles on the neck (see Chapter 6)
- Long Strokes (see Chapter 7)
- The Taffy Pull (see Chapters 5 and 7)
- Ankles Away (see Chapters 5 and 7)
- This Little Piggy (see Chapter 5)
- Raking (see Chapters 5 and 7)
- I Love You (see Chapter 5)
- Sun and Moon (see Chapter 5)
- The Heart Stroke (see Chapter 5)
- Alternating Hands (see Chapter 5)
- Thumb Circles on the wrists (see Chapter 5)
- Hand stroking (see Chapter 5)
- Finger stroking (see Chapter 5)
- Large Bottom Stroke (see Chapter 7)
- Long Effleurage Stroke (see Chapter 7)

In addition to massage, use the following tips to help your baby feel comforted:

- ✔ Swaddle your baby in a warm blanket (see Chapter 3).
- ✔ Wear your baby in a sling (see Chapter 1).
- ✔ Feed your baby often (at least every three hours).
- ✔ Introduce new things only when your baby is in a calm and relaxed state.
- ✔ When rocking your baby, move slowly and gently.
- ✔ Make gentle contact with your baby if she tends to space out. Use eye contact or a soft touch.

Sometimes even eye contact is too stimulating, especially with babies born addicted to cocaine.

Addressing fetal alcohol syndrome

Babies who suffer from severe effects of maternal alcohol use are diagnosed with fetal alcohol syndrome (FAS) — a lifelong and disabling syndrome. The Centers for Disease Control (CDC) estimate that as many as 3 out of 2,000 babies born in the United States have FAS.

The cause of FAS

Alcoholism is a serious problem in the United States. Alcohol abuse during pregnancy causes devastating results in babies and children. Despite our knowledge of the effects of alcohol on a fetus, as many as 1 in 30 pregnant women in the United States reports having seven or more drinks per week during pregnancy.

When a pregnant woman drinks, the alcohol enters her blood system, crosses the placenta, and is passed on to her fetus. In a fetus, the alcohol breaks down slowly. The alcohol stays in a fetus's body longer than in an adult's.

In the first three months of pregnancy, alcohol can cause the physical defects of FAS. During the second trimester, the mother is at risk of losing her baby to a miscarriage. And during the last trimester, severe growth deficiencies can occur.

Although there is no proven safe amount of alcohol that pregnant woman can consume, cases of FAS are usually seen in babies whose mothers are alcoholics or binge drinkers.

Symptoms

The effects of alcohol on a baby are severe and devastating. Three general areas of development are affected:

- ✔ **Facial appearance:** A baby with FAS usually has small eye openings, a small face, a short upturned nose, a flat mid-face, a wide nose bridge, and a thin upper lip. The FAS facial characteristics tend to become more normal-looking in adolescence. Babies with FAS are at risk for a cleft palate and underdeveloped jaw.

Even though many woman stop drinking during the first trimester (as soon as they learn they are pregnant), this is when the eyes develop. The eyes are the first facial feature to be affected, and the damage is irreversible.

- ✔ **Central nervous system:** Babies with FAS experience developmental delays (especially in balance and coordination) and decreased muscle strength. They usually experience tremors, and children with FAS have low intellectual functioning and skills. Some of the issues they suffer with include AD/HD, behavior problems, poor impulse control, and poor judgment. As they grow into children and young adults, they typically have difficulty forming relationships and suffer from other mental health problems.

Children with FAS can be unpredictable and impulsive. They often need 24-hour monitoring.

✔ **Growth:** Low birth weight is common among babies with FAS; so is less-than-average height and head circumference. Although the facial features of babies with FAS tend to change when they reach adolescence, the height and head circumference do not, and the measurements stay well below normal.

Although many of the obvious physical effects of FAS are no longer apparent in adulthood, the behavioral and cognitive problems are lifelong. FAS is the most common cause of mental retardation (see Chapter 12).

Treatment and healing

Because FAS is a permanent diagnosis, treatment options are limited. Some deformities can be changed with surgery, but others cannot. Psychotropic medication can help some behavioral and mental health issues.

The majority of babies and children with FAS are raised by relatives of the birth mother, foster parents, or adoptive families.

Helping babies diagnosed with FAS includes aiding in forming attachment with the caretakers, as well as either stimulating or calming the central nervous system. Massaging a baby with FAS can help you accomplish both.

It may be hard to identify a newborn with FAS. Withdrawal symptoms may not occur until the baby is home from the hospital. Also, many of the identifying characteristics do not show up until 2 to 3 years of age. If you are adopting or have a foster child whose mother has a history of alcoholism, you may want to assume the baby could have at least a mild case of FAS. Assuming the possibility of FAS at least ensures that you will carefully monitor the growth and development of your baby.

If your baby has been diagnosed with FAS, keep these things in mind:

✔ You want to practice attachment parenting and use as many of the attachment parenting tools as possible (see Chapter 1).

✔ Children with FAS seem to do well with families who are low key, quiet, and stable.

✔ You need to set consistent boundaries and serve as a role model.

Massage techniques for FAS

The goal of massage for FAS is to foster an attachment and to either calm or stimulate the central nervous system. You don't need to use any special stroke to foster an attachment; simply spending extra time touching and making contact with your baby will help you bond.

The nervous system is a different story: You need to be careful when choosing massage techniques to use because you want to tailor your touch to your baby's specific needs.

Stimulating the central nervous system

If your baby's nervous system is slow, you can use strokes to stimulate it. However, you don't want to risk overstimulating your baby, even if he has an underactive nervous system. As always, look for cues of overstimulation (see Chapter 4), and trust your intuition.

Here are some massage techniques you can use to stimulate the nervous system:

✔ Use *petrissage* strokes (which involve kneading, wringing, rolling, or squeezing), such as:

- Kneading Dough (see Chapters 5 and 7)
- Squeeze and Twist (see Chapters 5 and 7)
- Thumb Circles (see Chapters 5 and 7)
- The C Stroke (see Chapter 5)
- Alternating Thumbs (see Chapter 7)

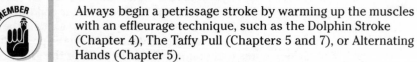 Always begin a petrissage stroke by warming up the muscles with an effleurage technique, such as the Dolphin Stroke (Chapter 4), The Taffy Pull (Chapters 5 and 7), or Alternating Hands (Chapter 5).

✔ Use abdominal or chest strokes (see Chapter 5).

✔ Alternate using strokes in an upward (stimulating) and downward (relaxing) flow.

✔ Massage your baby after a nap.

✔ Include games, rhymes, and music during your massage (see Chapter 9).

✔ Be sure to give your baby a massage during tummy time.

✔ Massage your baby at unexpected times, as well as during your daily routine. For example, massage your baby every morning after a nap and then several times throughout the day at the changing table.

✔ Use some of the massage techniques from Chapter 14 to add variety to your massage sequence.

Calming the central nervous system

If your baby has an overly sensitive nervous system, you need to practice techniques to soothe it. Here are some examples:

✔ Spend a lot of time holding and cuddling your baby before beginning to use any massage sequence. When your baby can tolerate touch, start introducing gentle massage strokes.

✔ In the beginning, introduce effleurage strokes one at a time:

- The Dolphin Stroke (see Chapter 4)
- The Taffy Pull (see Chapters 5 and 7)
- Raking (see Chapters 5 and 7)
- Alternating Hands (see Chapter 5)
- Hand stroking (see Chapter 5)
- Finger stroking (see Chapter 5)

✔ Massage your baby's face, but only if she enjoys it. Some babies love having their faces and heads touched and massaged. Others find it too stimulating. Watch your baby's cues, and stop if it becomes too stimulating for her. Some techniques (from Chapter 6) to try include:

- The Smile Stroke
- Circling the Eyes
- The Open Book Stroke
- The Ear Stroke
- Chinny Chin Chin

✔ Use strokes in a downward direction only.

✔ Be sure to give the massage in a dark and quiet room.

✔ Give your baby a massage after a bath.

✔ Massage your baby with one hand while you are holding him.

✔ See Chapter 9 for our recommendations on how to handle temper tantrums.

Caring for the caregiver

Parenting a child with FAS means providing constant supervision, setting boundaries, getting medical care for the baby, finding financial help, and working with outside agencies to make sure your baby receives the proper intervention. It can be exhausting. Be sure to join a support group, ask for help when you need it, and keep realistic expectations.

The National Organization of Fetal Alcohol Syndrome (NOFAS) offers a listing of community support groups and resources in the United States. Contact NOFAS at 202-785-4585, or visit www.nofas.org.

Babies Exposed to HIV

The good news is that a pregnant mother who is HIV-positive can give birth to a baby who is HIV-negative, if she carefully follows specific procedures. The bad news is that many women still pass on HIV to their babies.

Assuming the mother follows the procedures she should, after the baby is born he needs to receive vaccinations, medication, and testing to ensure that he remains HIV-negative.

Many babies whose mothers are HIV-positive also cope with other issues from the time they are born, such as drug or alcohol addiction or placement in foster care or an adoptive family. Using compassionate touch and massage can help these babies navigate all these transitions more successfully.

Navigating pregnancy with HIV

When a pregnant woman has HIV, she will most likely pass on the virus to her baby unless she follows certain protocols. HIV can be passed on to babies during pregnancy, during delivery, or through breastfeeding. Most incidences of HIV transmission occur during labor.

The medication that an HIV-positive mother and her baby need to take to prevent transmission of the virus could possibly have serious side effects. Doctors and researchers don't yet know the extent of the side effects because of the relatively short time they have been providing treatment and prevention.

Steps to prevent transmission

An HIV-positive mother may continue to take her HIV drugs or stop her medication early in the pregnancy and restart it later during pregnancy. If she is newly diagnosed with HIV, she may consider waiting until the second trimester to begin medication.

HIV, AIDS, and women

The Centers for Disease Control estimates that 280 to 370 children are born with HIV each year in the United States. Here are some other disturbing statistics regarding women, babies, HIV, and AIDS, pulled from the Elizabeth Glaser Pediatric Aids Foundation Web site (`www.pedaids.org`):

✔ Worldwide, 50 percent of all people now living with HIV or AIDS are women.

✔ Ninety-one percent of children who are HIV-positive in the United States got the virus from their mothers.

✔ AIDS is the leading cause of death for African American women ages 25 to 34.

✔ Worldwide, approximately 2,000 children are infected with HIV every day.

✔ An estimated 13 million children have been orphaned due to AIDS.

Certain HIV medications are known not to be safe to take during pregnancy:

✔ Efavirenz

✔ D4T

✔ ddI and d4t combined

✔ Amprenavir (oral liquid)

✔ Hydroxyurea

Assuming the mother is taking medications other than those listed above, the reason for not taking medication during part of the pregnancy is that the effects of other HIV medications on a fetus are largely unknown. Because transmission of HIV usually occurs late in pregnancy, the mother may opt to reduce potential risks to the fetus by stopping her medication for a short time.

An HIV-positive mother should talk with her doctor about taking an antiviral medication like AZT, which, if taken during the last six months of pregnancy, reduces the transmission rate to about 4 percent. So far, birth defects and long-term side effects to the fetus from AZT use during pregnancy have not been observed.

Even more effective than taking AZT during pregnancy is following a short course of treatment during labor and delivery that combines drugs like Nevirapine and AZT. Using this treatment reduces the transmission rate to 1 to 2 percent.

However, taking HIV medications during the pregnancy can affect how successful the later treatments (if needed) will be for both the mother and baby, if the virus develops a resistance to the medication.

The mother can also take other steps to help ensure that HIV will not be transmitted to her baby, including:

✔ Maintaining excellent prenatal care

✔ Exercising

✔ Not smoking

✔ Getting adequate rest

✔ Scheduling a C section (to avoid the baby coming in contact with the mother's blood during delivery)

However, women with a *low viral load* who are taking a combination of medications can have a vaginal birth. What is a low viral load? Viral load tests measure the progression of HIV in the body by testing the amount of the virus in the blood. Infants born to HIV-positive mothers test positive for HIV antibodies in a viral load test until 12 to 18 months of age because they carry their mothers' antibodies. Mothers with higher viral loads are more likely to infect their babies than those with low viral loads.

✔ Feeding the baby formula. Although controversy exists regarding breastfeeding, the current recommendation in the United States is that the safest way to avoid infection after birth is not to breastfeed.

In developing countries, where clean water is an issue, breastfeeding is considered the better choice. Even though the risk of infecting the baby is serious, the effects of drinking contaminated water are more serious.

HIV tests

Standard HIV tests detect the presence of antibodies that fight HIV; they do not detect the presence of HIV itself. Because babies carry their mothers' antibodies until approximately 18 months, a baby whose mother has HIV may test positive for the virus shortly after birth, even if he is not infected. For this reason, it may not be possible to determine whether a baby has been infected with HIV until he has reached 18 months of age. Babies who are infected with HIV continue to test positive beyond 18 months.

A different kind of test — the polymerase chain reaction (PCR) test — actually looks for HIV in the body, not antibodies. The preferred method of testing is to offer a first PCR test 48 hours after delivery and, if it is positive, to retest at 14 days. This procedure helps achieve an earlier diagnosis.

Why doesn't everyone get the PCR test? Whether you are offered a standard HIV test or a PCR test may be determined by where you live. The PCR test is expensive, requires the healthcare provider to have specialized training, and is labor-intensive.

Symptoms of HIV-positive babies

Babies with HIV may begin showing flu-like symptoms within a month of birth. Other signs of HIV may start to become evident at around 6 months of age, including:

- Slow growth and lack of weight gain
- Yeast infections
- Severe diaper rash
- Developmental delays
- Neurological problems

Severe symptoms, such as chronic diarrhea or lung disease, may not appear until the baby is 2 years old.

 Due to poor immune functioning, HIV-positive babies are at risk for catching the flu and other illnesses. In particular, the herpes virus *cytomegalovirus* (CMV) can be deadly to HIV-positive babies. Most healthy people come in contact with CMV and experience few or no symptoms. But babies with compromised immune systems may come down with pneumonia, stunted brain growth, and other severe problems. There seems to be some interplay between HIV and CMV: Babies with HIV catch CMV more easily, and some researchers believe that CMV may contain a protein that helps HIV spread.

Symptoms of CMV are:

- Lung problems
- Growth and developmental delays
- Dental abnormalities
- Poor weight gain
- Swollen glands
- Hepatitis
- Blood problems

As with HIV, many babies do not show symptoms of CMV right away. However, premature babies may show symptoms early.

Massaging babies with (or exposed to) HIV

The massage treatment for babies exposed to HIV and babies who have the virus is the same. HIV-exposed babies are placed on medication to prevent the transmission of the virus, even though they may be HIV-negative. These babies are under stress and affected by the medication just as babies with HIV are.

Massage benefits HIV-positive babies in the following ways:

✔ It improves immune system functioning.

✔ It increases relaxation hormones.

✔ It promotes weight gain.

✔ It helps the baby sleep.

✔ It increases the baby's attachment with the caregiver.

✔ It positively affects intellectual developmental.

Babies who may not have the virus but are taking HIV medication preventatively receive the following benefits from massage:

✔ It increases their relaxation hormones.

✔ It helps babies under stress to sleep better.

✔ It creates a bond between the baby and the caregiver.

There aren't any particular massage strokes or techniques that you need to use to help your baby. Generally, you can choose any of the strokes or sequences we list throughout the book. However, here are a few tips to keep in mind:

✔ Babies typically begin taking medications like AZT right after birth. The type of medication they take depends upon what medication the mother was taking during pregnancy. Drugs like AZT can have serious side effects to the baby, such as anemia or congestive heart failure. If your baby experiences such side effects, check with your healthcare provider about strokes you would like to use to be sure there aren't any contraindications.

✔ Potent medications may make your baby ill in other ways as well; diarrhea and vomiting are common side effects. If your baby is sick from medication, holding and cuddling will be enough initially. You need to wait to introduce a massage sequence.

✔ Stability and consistency are very important to the health of these babies. You can use massage to create a routine of nurturing, loving touch.

Babies often have to take medication three or four times a day. In order to help them take the medication, a routine must be established. You could help make the routine a little nicer by rewarding taking the medication with a nurturing massage afterwards.

✔ HIV-positive babies often have associated illnesses that may affect their health. Some of these illnesses and conditions could be:

- Cardiovascular problems
- Behavioral problems
- Anemia

Less severe conditions, such as chronic sinusitis and digestive troubles, can be eased with massage techniques (see Chapter 11).

✔ Some infants and children get headaches as a side effect of medications. Following is a massage sequence just for headaches:

- The Dolphin Stroke (see Chapter 4)
- Ears to Chin (see Chapter 6)
- Circling the Eyes (see Chapter 6)
- The Open Book Stroke (see Chapters 5 and 6)
- Big Circles (see Chapter 6)
- The Temple Stroke (see Chapter 6)
- Long Strokes (see Chapter 7)

If your baby won't tolerate a whole massage sequence just yet, try only one or two strokes. Good choices would be The Open Book and Temple strokes.

Be sure to include the neck and shoulders in your headache massage. Tension held here could contribute to a headache.

Finish your headache relief massage by holding onto your baby's feet for a few moments and breathing. Imagine you can feel your baby's energy moving down through her body to her feet.

✔ Many HIV-positive babies' lives are in transition; they may be waiting for permanent home placements. Massage techniques and tips from Chapter 12 may be helpful.

The majority of babies diagnosed with HIV — about 80 percent — experience a slow progression of the disease and show very few symptoms as they grow older. About 20 percent of babies diagnosed with HIV become very ill within their first year and have a short life expectancy. Factors that determine how the disease progresses include how early the diagnosis was given and the type of care the baby received.

Using other complementary therapies

The term *complementary therapy* refers to therapies that complement traditional treatments. Massage therapy is typically considered a complementary therapy (as well as a preventative therapy because regular massage can prevent many stress-related illnesses).

In addition to massage, you can use other complementary therapies along with traditional treatments to maintain the health of your HIV-positive baby. Some of these therapies are:

✔ Acupuncture, which we discuss in Chapter 11

✔ CranioSacral Therapy, which we also discuss in Chapter 11

✔ Nutrition and vitamin therapy, which you can research online at sites such as www.hivresources.com and www.doctor yourself.com

✔ Baby yoga, which you can read about at www.itsybitsy yoga.com

✔ Chiropractic care, which we explain in Chapter 7

 Always let your regular healthcare provider know when you are using complementary therapies.

Taking universal precautions

Using universal precautions prevents contact with the HIV virus. While it is important for you to touch and massage your baby, you must also protect yourself, other caregivers, and family members from the virus. We recommend that you read the following list and use your judgment as to what precautions are right for your family and situation.

We realize that the following suggestions seem very clinical. We do think they are important, however, because practicing universal precautions is a reality when a loved one has HIV or AIDS.

> ✔ Use barrier protection (such as gloves) if there is a potential of your skin coming in contact with the baby's blood.
>
> ✔ Wash your hands (or other body parts) immediately and thoroughly if they come in contact with the baby's blood.
>
> ✔ Do everything possible to avoid your baby having accidental injuries. Keep sharp objects well out of reach, for example.

Additional Resources

Drug or alcohol addiction and HIV/AIDS are serious issues that affect families in profound ways. Adding baby massage to your routine will no doubt help you and your baby significantly. However, you still need a ton of support.

We have included this resource list in the hope that having access to additional information, support, and community resources puts you in a stronger position to help your family.

For babies affected by drug and alcohol addiction

Following are lists of organizations, books, and videos that are related to addictions.

Institutes and centers

The following organizations offer information, referrals, and support regarding the effects of drugs on babies.

National Dissemination Center for Children with Disabilities (NICHCY)

The NICHCY offers information on disabilities in infants, toddlers, and children. They offer a state-by-state listing of resources in the United States.

P.O. Box 1492
Washington, DC 20013
Phone: 800-695-0285 (v/tty)
Fax: 202-884-8441
Web: nichcy@aed.org

FAS Family Resource Institute

FAS provides referrals, support, training, and workshops to families and individuals affected by fetal alcohol syndrome.

P.O. Box 2525
Lynnwood, WA 98036
E-mail: vicky@fetalalcoholsyndrome.org

The National Toxicology Program (NTP) Center for the Evaluation of Risks to Human Reproduction (CERHR)

The NTP offers the latest information regarding the effects of chemicals and drugs on development and reproduction.

Dr. Michael D. Shelby
NIEHS EC-32
P.O. Box 12233
Research Triangle Park, NC 27709
Phone: 919-541-3455
Fax: 919-316-4511
E-mail: shelby@niehs.nih.gov

Families Anonymous

Families Anonymous is a 12-step program that offers support groups for family members of the person with the substance abuse problem. The substance abuser does not attend meetings.

P.O. Box 3475
Culver City, CA 90231
800-736-9805 or 310-815-8010
E-mail: Famanon@familiesanonymous.org
Web: www.familiesanonymous.org

Do It Now Foundation

The Do It Now Foundation offers information on the effects of alcoholism and drug abuse on fetuses and babies.

P.O. Box 27568
Tempe, AZ 85285
480-736-0599
Web: www.doitnow.org

Books and videos

The following books and videos offer practical information on healing from addictions while pregnant and parenting a baby or child with special needs:

✔ *When Your Child Has a Disability: The Complete Sourcebook of Daily and Medical Care* (Paul H. Brookes Publishing), edited by Mark L. Batshaw. Go to www.brookespublishing.com.

✔ *The Mother's Survival Guide to Recovery: All About Alcohol, Drugs & Babies* (New Harbinger Publications) by Laurie Tanner.

✔ *A Woman's Addiction Workbook: Your Guide to In-Depth Healing* (New Harbinger Publications) by Lisa M. Najavits.

✔ *Successfully Parenting Your Baby with Special Needs: Early Intervention for Ages Birth to Three* (video, Paul H. Brookes Publishing), produced by Grace M. Hanlon. Go to www.brookespublishing.com.

For babies and children affected by HIV and AIDS

The following sections list associations and informational resources on HIV, AIDS, and babies.

Foundations and organizations

The following foundations and organizations fund research, provide referrals, and help to find families for babies affected by HIV/AIDS.

Children With AIDS Project of America (CWA)

The CWA recruits families to adopt babies and children who are HIV-positive, AIDS orphans, or born drug-addicted. They also offer advocacy and support.

P.O. Box 23778
Tempe, AZ 85285-3778
Phone: 480-774-9718
Fax: 480-921-0449
Web: www.aidskids.org

The Firelight Foundation

The Firelight Foundation offers grants that support the needs and rights of children orphaned or affected by AIDS in Sub-Saharan Africa.

510 Mission Street
Santa Cruz, CA 95060
Phone: 831-429-8750
Web: www.firelightfoundation.org

Elizabeth Glaser Pediatric AIDS Foundation

The Elizabeth Glaser Pediatric AIDS Foundation offers referrals, resources, and grants to help eradicate pediatric AIDS.

Contact Chris Hudnall, Resource Coordinator, at 310-314-1459 ext. 154 or chris@pedaids.org for family referrals to find the best care.

2950 31st Street #125
Santa Monica, CA 90405
Web: www.pedaids.org

Mind/Body Institute

The Mind/Body Institute offers a medical clinic for HIV- and AIDS-related disorders. The focus of the treatments is on the relaxation response, cognitive-behavioral strategies for coping, nutrition, and light exercise.

824 Bolyston Street
Chestnut Hill, MA 02467
Phone: 617-991-0112

Web sites

These two Web sites provide a wealth of information about HIV and AIDS:

- ✔ www.aids.org: This Web site provides prevention, testing, and treatment information regarding AIDS and HIV.

- ✔ www.The Body.com: This up-to-date Web site offers information on 550 topics related to AIDS and HIV.

Books

The following books offer information, insights, and practical help to women and families dealing with HIV and AIDS:

- ✔ *Troubling the Angels: Women Living with HIV/AIDS* (Westview Press) by Patricia Ann Lather and Chris Smithies

- ✔ *Children and HIV/AIDS* (Transaction Publishers) by Gary Anderson, Constance Ryan, Susan Taylor-Brown, and Myra White-Gray

- ✔ *Nutrition and HIV: A New Model for Treatment* (Jossey-Bass) by Mary Romeyn

- ✔ *HIV and AIDS in Mothers and Babies: A Guide to Counseling* (Mosby-Year Book, Inc.) by Lorraine Sherr

Part V
The Part of Tens

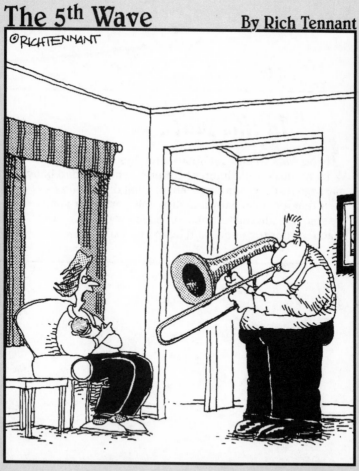

"Y'know, I think some oil and a little soothing music are all we need."

In this part . . .

1 f you want to find out about stretches and massage techniques from different cultures, where to find baby massage resources on the Web, or what organizations exist that focus on baby massage, this part is for you. We also include suggestions for videos you can use to practice your technique and learn new skills.

Chapter 14

(Almost) Ten Special Techniques

In This Chapter

▶ Exploring massages from other cultures

▶ Helping your baby stretch and sit tall

▶ Introducing your baby to yoga

*I*f you want to spice up your baby massage routine, this chapter is for you. We include massage techniques from other cultures, stretches, techniques to assist your baby's posture, and more. Have fun!

Trying Massages from Other Parts of the World

Infant massage is practiced in many cultures throughout the world. In this section, we offer just a sampling of the variety of massage techniques used.

Indian massage

This type of massage is based on Ayurvedic philosophy. First, a bit of background: *Ayurveda* (meaning "the knowledge of life") seeks harmony by balancing the body's energies through diet, exercise, yoga, and massage. The body's three energies are called *Vata*, *Pitta*, and *Kapha*. Each of us has all three energies, but we usually have one or two predominant ones. Ayurveda teaches how to balance these energies by appreciating and working with our body's true nature.

Followers of Ayurvedic philosophy give their newborns a daily massage before their bath. The massage consists of dipping a soft wheat dough ball in almond oil (along with a dash of turmeric) and rolling the ball along the infant's back (lengthwise). The purpose of the infant massage is to energetically cleanse and to increase circulation, eliminate toxins, and assist in digestion.

When the newborn is a month old, the baby's daily massage changes. The focus of this massage is on the muscle groups used to support the body (in the back, neck, abdomen, arms, and legs).

In Indian culture, massage is recommended for babies until approximately 2 years of age. You can find more information on this type of massage by reading *Ayurvedic Massage: Traditional Indian Techniques for Balancing Body and Mind* by Harish Johari (Healing Arts Press).

Tui Na massage

Like acupuncture (which we discuss in Chapter 12), Tui Na massage (Chinese massage) works by balancing the body's energy, called *Oi*. Unlike acupuncture, it doesn't use needles!

Chinese massage is touted as an excellent remedy for colic and fussiness. People who use this type of massage believe that a baby's energy channels (called *meridians*) can be affected by the many developmental changes that occur from infancy through childhood. They believe that balancing your baby's flow of energy adds harmony to the body and lessens the effects of blocked energy flow.

If your baby is restless, try using the following Tui Na stroke on his forehead:

1. **Place both thumbs on their sides with your fingertips facing each other in the center of your baby's forehead, just above the middle of his eyebrows.**

2. **Use slight pressure and move one thumb up towards the hairline, immediately followed by your other thumb.**

3. **Use this same motion — one thumb stroking up toward the hairline, followed by the other — for a few minutes.**

Because your baby is restless when you start this treatment, he may become slightly more restless or agitated when you begin and then show signs of calming down.

If you want to find out more about Chinese Massage, read *The Handbook of Chinese Massage: Tui Na Techniques to Awaken Body and Mind,* by Maria Mercati (Healing Arts Press).

Shiatsu massage

Shiatsu is a form of Japanese massage. It is similar to Chinese (Tui Na) massage in that pressure points are stimulated in order to balance energy. What makes Shiatsu unique is the addition of lifts, twists, and stretches to the massage sequence.

You can add a simple Shiatsu technique to your repertoire by using the following leg stretch:

1. **Lay your baby on her belly.**

2. **Place one hand on her *sacrum*. (See Figure 7-12 in Chapter 7 to see where the sacrum is located.)**

3. **Lift and bend both of your baby's legs to bring her feet in towards the buttocks.**

4. **Apply gentle, downward pressure onto your baby's lower back.**

African massage

In some African cultures, babies are massaged with hot compresses to relax their muscles. You can do this at home by running a washcloth under water that is not too hot, rolling it into a ball, and gently pressing it onto your baby's body.

Keep the unmassaged parts of your baby's body covered so she stays warm.

Stretching

Generally speaking, stretching is good for everyone. It relaxes your muscles, reduces stress, and increases flexibility. You don't really have to teach your baby to stretch, because babies do it naturally. However, you can incorporate assisted stretches into your massage routine. In this section, we show you how.

Arm stretches

Stretching your newborn's arms helps to relieve stress and lengthen unused muscles. Older babies love it just because it feels good.

The Arm Cross is an easy stretch to incorporate into your massage routine:

1. **While your baby is lying on her back, take hold of her right arm and pull the arm gently across her chest toward the opposite side of her body.**

2. **As you are pulling the right arm across her chest, simultaneously pull her left arm gently across her chest toward the opposite side of her body (see Figure 14-1).**

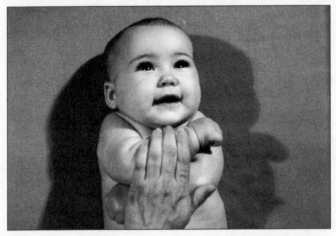

Figure 14-1: Simultaneously stretch both arms across your baby's body.

Leg stretches

You can assist your baby as he develops muscle strength in his legs by including stretches in your massage.

Use the Leg Cross stretch during your regular massage or even on the changing table. Here's how:

1. **Cross your baby's lower legs.**

2. **Gently push both knees toward his chest, making sure to keep his bottom on the floor, bed, or table (see Figure 14-2).**

3. **Cross your baby's legs the other way, and repeat Step 2.**

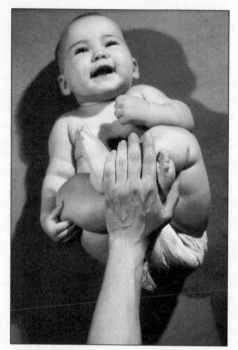

Figure 14-2: Gently push both legs toward your baby's chest.

Helping Your Baby's Posture

You can help your baby protect her developing spine by supporting her when she is learning to sit. In this section, we show you how.

Supported sitting

When babies are first learning to sit, they slump and slouch and wind up sitting more on the spine than their legs. You can help your baby's spine by gently pulling her body forward a bit and placing her hands on the floor in front of her. Watch her spine lengthen into its natural curve.

Even if your baby looks secure in this posture, stay close by to catch her in case she topples over.

Unsupported sitting

After your baby has mastered sitting, you can help keep her hips open by spreading her legs a little wider than usual in front of her. Push her forward slightly, and use this opportunity to give her back and neck a massage.

Even babies who can sit by themselves tend to slide down and slouch when they get tired. Keep an eye on your baby's posture; if she slides down onto her lower back, she may need a nap or a change of scenery.

Bringing Baby into Your Yoga Routine

If you practice yoga, you're in luck! When you bring your baby into your yoga routine, you are able to spend quality time relaxing and bonding with your little one physically, emotionally, spiritually, and energetically. Of course, babies aren't able to practice the postures on their own, but get creative and find ways to bring your baby into your yoga postures — see Figure 14-3 for an example.

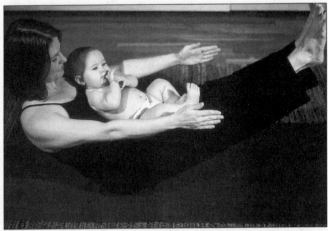

Figure 14-3: Let your little one mold to your body in *Navasana* (Boat Pose).

In Chapter 15, we recommend a video on postnatal yoga that offers lots of great ideas for making your baby part of your yoga routine.

Chapter 15

Ten Great Massage Resources

In This Chapter

▶ Finding resources online

▶ Locating great organizations

▶ Watching useful videos

*I*f this book has piqued your curiosity and you're interested in finding out even more about baby massage, you're in luck — you have a variety of resources to choose from. In this chapter, we direct you toward some of our favorite sources of information, including Web sites, organizations, and videos.

Surfing the Web

A plethora of baby massage-related information is available online. Following are some of our picks for the most useful Web sites to visit.

www.InfantMassage.com

You can find virtually everything you need to know about infant massage on this Web site. It includes a directory of infant massage classes available in your area, and if you are a massage practitioner, you can become a certified Premature Infant Massage Instructor through this site's program.

www.AskDrSears.com

Dr. Bill and Martha Sears, along with two of their sons (who are pediatricians), offer information on this site about baby massage, attachment parenting, co-sleeping, nursing, and the basics of sensitive parenting and childcare.

www.HealthyFamily.org

A Foundation for Healthy Family Living (AFHFL) offers infant massage education and training to parents, families, hospitals, and interested organizations. We like this foundation because it is dedicated to creating healthy families and communities through education about respectful communication and nurturing touch.

www.LittleForest.com

Did you know that some baby lotions contain formaldehyde and some tearless shampoos contain numbing agents? That's why Little Forest creates 100 percent natural baby products that you can use to massage and bathe your baby. This company has an extensive list of products that you can purchase online.

Finding Massage Associations

Following are several associations that you can contact if you'd like to know more about massage or body work.

American Massage Therapy Association

The American Massage Therapy Association (AMTA) exists to advance the practice of massage therapy, set ethical standards, and promote health. This organization is located in Evanston, Illinois. You can reach its offices at 847-864-0123 or contact AMTA online at www.AMTAmassage.org.

International Association of Infant Massage

We introduce you to the International Association of Infant Massage (IAIM) in Chapter 1. This organization is located in Ventura, California and can be reached at 805-644-8524 or by visiting the Web site at www.iaim-us.com.

International Loving Touch Foundation

The International Loving Touch Foundation (ILTF) offers training programs for infant massage instructors and information on where to find one in your area. You can also order books, videos, oils, and music from its Web site, www.lovingtouch.com. ILTF is located in Portland, Oregon and can be reached at 502-253-8482.

Associated Bodywork & Massage Professionals

Associated Bodywork & Massage Professionals (ABMP) is similar to the American Massage Therapy Association in that it offers resources and support for massage and bodywork professionals. We really like the magazine this organization publishes, *Massage and Bodywork,* and think it's worth the membership fee just for the subscription. The ABMP is located in Colorado and can be reached at 800-458-2267 or online at www.abmp.com.

Using Videos

The following videos are useful in helping you to learn new techniques and bring your baby into your yoga or exercise routines. They can all be purchased at www.FitnessBeginnings.com.

Baby Massage and Exercise

This video gives you easy and clear instructions to follow. The massage sequence is relaxing and nice to use just before bedtime.

Infant Massage/Postnatal Yoga Combo Pack

This video combination pack includes the hour-long *Infant Massage* video, which shows you some basics, as well as techniques to help with colic, gas, and other common ailments, in an easy-to-follow format.

Yoga Journal's Postnatal Yoga video, which also comes in this combo pack, is almost perfect for new moms wanting to start their postpartum yoga practice safely. Our only issue is that it is an hour long, and most new mothers don't have that much time! Several props are recommended for the sequences in this video: a blanket, block, mat, bolster, and chair.

Exercise with Daddy & Me

We include this video because it's a great way to encourage fathers to massage, stretch, and exercise with their babies. This 45-minute videotape was designed by a nurse and a pediatrician, and it contains warm-ups, exercises, cool-downs, and massage techniques.

Index

• A •

abdominal massage
  cautions, 54
  constipation relief, 181
  five-minute massage, 175
  I Love You stroke, 75–76
  Let's Go sequence, 166, 167
  overview, 72
  Sleeper sequence, 164
  Sun and Moon technique, 74–75
  Thumbs to Sides technique, 73–74
  Water Wheel technique, 72–73
acupuncture, 100, 213
addiction, 219–228
adhesion, 13
adopted baby, 201–204, 206, 216
adrenaline, 23–24
African massage, 243
ailment. *See also specific ailments*
  abdominal massage, 72
  benefits of massage, 16–17
  chest massage, 77
  Down syndrome complications, 210, 211
  endorphins, 18
  injured baby, 55
airplane, 176
alcohol, 36, 214, 219–228
alertness, 27–28, 141
All You Need Is Love: Beatles Songs for Kids (music CD), 149
allergy
  asthma causes, 184
  breastfeeding benefits, 142
  colic causes, 182
  oil, 51
Alternating Thumbs technique, 112–113

Amby Baby Motion Bed, 183
American Massage Therapy Association, 248
amino acid, 24
Anderson, Gary (*Children with HIV/AIDS*), 238
Ankles Away technique, 68–69, 112
ANS (autonomic nervous system), 23
anterior fontanel, 88
antibiotics, 100
apathy, 9
Apgar test, 139
arched back, 24
Are You My Mother? (Eastman, P.D.), 150
Arm Cross stretch, 243–244
arm massage
  "C" Stroke, 81–82
  five-minute massage, 175
  Little Sleeper sequence, 164–165
  overview, 81
  Sleeper sequence, 164
  Thumb Circles technique, 83
aromatherapy, 53, 56
ascending colon, 72
Asian culture, 17
Associated Bodywork & Massage Professionals, 249
asthma, 184–186
athetoid cerebral palsy, 211
attachment. *See also* bonding
  developmental delays, 207
  drug-addicted baby, 221
  fetal alcohol syndrome, 225
  overview, 199–200
  patterns, 200–201
  quality, 201
  reactive attachment disorder, 205–206

attachment parenting
  benefits, 10
  overview, 9
  sibling rivalry, 217
  tools, 9
attention
  older infants, 145–146
  overview, 14–15
  trust, 21
attunement, 32
autism, 214
autonomic nervous system
    (ANS), 23
awareness, 14–15
*Ayurvedic Massage: Traditional
    Indian Techniques for
    Balancing Body and Mind*
    (Johari, Harish), 242
ayurvedic philosophy, 241–242
AZT (medication), 229, 232

• *B* •

babbling, 146
baby. *See* infant
Baby Bjorn (front carrier), 120
baby oil, 51
baby wearing, 15, 120
baby wipe warmer, 173
babysitter, 42
Back and Forth technique, 119–120
back, arched, 24
back massage
  Back and Forth technique, 119–120
  buttocks, 112–116
  congestion relief, 190–191
  feet, 108
  five-minute massage, 175–176
  legs, 108–112
  Let's Go sequence, 166, 167
  Long Effleurage Stroke, 118–119
  neck, 126–127
  overstimulation, 118
  overview, 107–108

premature baby, 137
  raking, 125–126
  Sacral Stroke, 124–125
  shoulders, 126–127
  Sleeper sequence, 164
  Small Circles technique, 122–123
  Swooping technique, 121–122
bathing
  newborn guidelines, 169–171
  older infant guidelines, 171–172
  overview, 168
  safety, 169
  skin problems, 196, 197
Batshaw, Mark L. (*When Your Child
    Has a Disability: The Complete
    Sourcebook of Daily and
    Medical Care*), 236
*Beauty and the Beast: Original
    Motion Picture Soundtrack*
    (music CD), 149
bed, 50
belly. *See* abdominal massage
Big Circles technique, 96–99
biting, 187, 188
blanket, 34–35, 134, 167
blood test, 139
body language, 39, 42
bonding. *See also* attachment
  adopted baby, 201–204
  attachment parenting, 9–11
  baby wearing, 15
  benefits of massage, 19–21
  depression, 27
  fathers, 12
  hormone, 20
  hospital stay, 19–20, 34, 136
  importance of touch, 8–11
  kangaroo care, 136
  oil application steps, 56
  overview, 19–20
  premature baby, 133, 134
  siblings, 151
  tips, 20

books
  addiction topics, 236–237
  children's, 149–150
  HIV and AIDS, 238
boredom, 39–40
boundaries, 154–155
brain development, 28–29
breast cancer, 142
breastfeeding
  adopted baby, 202
  asthma, 185
  during bath, 170
  benefits, 142
  cold prevention, 191
  constipation, 180
  gas, 72
  HIV-infected mother, 230
  massage benefits, 20
  massage incorporation, 141–143
  past view of, 8
  premature baby, 134, 142
  resources, 202
  SIDS prevention, 167
  skin problems, 196
  teething, 188
Breastfeeding For Dummies
      (Perkins, Sharon and
      Vannais, Carol), 72
breathing
  asthma, 184–186
  chest massage, 76
  co-sleeping, 36
  crying baby, 16
  grounding technique, 141
  intention, 15
  massage preparation, 47–48
  stress, 25, 184
broken bone, 55
Brown, Margaret Wise (*Goodnight
      Moon*), 150
Butterfly Stroke, 79–80
buttocks, 112–116, 137

• C •

"C" Stroke, 81–82
Caesarean delivery, 8, 230
car seat, 171
car travel, 176
central nervous system,
      224, 226–227
cerebral palsy (CP), 211–213
cervical spine, 116
changing table, 172–174
cheeks, 91–92
chest congestion, 189–191, 211
chest massage
  Butterfly Stroke, 79–80
  five-minute massage, 175
  Heart Stroke, 77–78
  Let's Go sequence, 166, 167
  Open Book Stroke, 78–79
  overview, 76
childbirth
  baby wearing, 15
  drugs, 221
  importance of touch, 8–9
  natural delivery, 139
  routine tests, 139
Children With AIDS Project of
      America (nonprofit
      organization), 237
Children with HIV/AIDS (Anderson,
      Gary, Ryan, Constance,
      Taylor-Brown, Susan, and
      White-Gray, Myra), 238
Chinese medicine
  foot massage, 69
  hand containment, 135
  immune system, 29
Chinny Chin Chin technique,
      102–104
chiropractic care, 100, 124
chromosomal abnormality, 208–209
Circling the Eyes technique, 93–94

Circular Palmer technique, 113–114
circulation
  goal of massage, 13
  Kneading Dough technique, 65
  premature baby, 15
classical music, 51
clothing
  baby with Down syndrome, 211
  bathing tips, 169, 171
  diaper change massage, 173
  massage preparation, 55–56
  massaging through, 35
  overstimulation, 140
  skin problems, 197
CMV (cytomegalovirus), 231
cocaine-exposed baby, 12
cold, 189–190
colicky baby. *See also* crying baby
  benefits of massage, 16
  cause of colic, 182
  Chinese massage, 242
  compassion of parent, 30
  endorphins, 18
  onset of colic, 37
  overview, 181–182
  stress, 184
  techniques for relief, 182–183
colon, 72–76
communication, 21, 134, 215
complementary therapy, 234. *See also specific types*
confidence, 21–22
congestion, 189–191, 211
consistency, 154, 233
constipation, 179–181, 213
contractures, 213
corrected age, 138
cortisol, 23–24
co-sleeping, 36, 167, 203
CP (cerebral palsy), 211–213
cradle cap, 197–198
CranioSacral Therapy, 213
crawling, 41, 146
crib, 36

crying baby. *See also* colicky baby
  breathing techniques, 16
  compassion of parent, 30
  emotional development, 35, 37
  first massage, 56
  meaning of cries, 37
  overstimulation signs, 54
  signs of stress, 24
  spoiled child, 10–11
culture, 204
cupping, 213
curiosity, 148
cytomegalovirus (CMV), 231

• *D* •

depression, 12, 26–27
descending colon, 72, 75
detachment, 9, 14
development. *See* infant development
diaper
  change, 161, 172–174
  massage preparation, 55–56
diaphragmatic breathing, 26
diffuser, 53
digestion
  abdominal massage, 72
  benefits of massage, 28
  effects of stress, 28
  solid foods, 180
  timing of massage, 54
The Discipline Book: How to Have a Better-Behaved Child from Birth to Age Ten (Sears, William and Sears, Martha), 156
Do It Now Foundation (nonprofit organization), 236
Dolphin Stroke, 56–59
Down syndrome, 208–211
drooling, 187
drug-addicted baby, 219–228, 235–237

• E •

ear infection, 100
Ear Stroke, 101–102
Ears to Chin technique, 88–89
Eastman, P.D. (*Are You My Mother?*), 150
eczema, 196–197
effleurage stroke
  Alternating Hands technique, 81
  definition, 12
  fetal alcohol syndrome, 227
  Long Effleurage Stroke, 118–119
  Taffy Pull, 64
Elizabeth Glaser Pediatric AIDS Foundation, 238
emotional development
  attunement, 32
  fussy baby, 34, 37
  hospital stay, 34
  overstimulation, 32–33
  person permanence, 41
  play, 38, 39–40
  relationship building, 38
  schedule, 33–34, 36–37
  touch, 35
endorphin, 18, 139
energy medicine, 3
epidural, 8, 221
essential oil, 53, 191
eucalyptus oil, 191
Eustachian tube, 100
expressions, 39
eye contact
  benefits, 21
  drug-addicted baby, 223
  overstimulation, 54
  premature baby, 137
  readiness cues, 46
eye ointment, 139
eyes, 93–94, 224

• F •

facial massage
  Big Circles technique, 96–99
  cautions, 87–88
  Chinny Chin Chin technique, 102–104
  Circling the Eyes technique, 93–94
  congestion relief, 191
  Ear Stroke, 101–102
  Ears to Chin technique, 88–89
  fetal alcohol syndrome, 227
  Open Book Stroke, 94–96
  Sleeper sequence, 164
  Small Circles technique, 89–90
  Smile Stroke, 91–92
  Tapping the Jaw Line, 90–91
  Temple Stroke, 99, 101
failure to thrive syndrome, 138
faith, 17
Families Anonymous (substance abuse recovery program), 236
family, 27, 150–152
FAS Family Resource Institute, 236
FAS (fetal alcohol syndrome)
  caregiver support, 227–228
  cause, 224
  massage techniques, 226–227
  overview, 223
  resources, 235–237
  symptoms, 224–225
  treatment, 225
fascia, 13
father
  benefits of massage, 22
  bonding, 12
  exercise video, 250
  fetal alcohol syndrome support, 228
  frustration with colicky baby, 184
  high need baby tips, 195
  kangaroo care, 136
  postpartum depression, 27
  resources for support, 35

fatigue, 143
fetal alcohol syndrome (FAS).
    See FAS
fever, 55, 187
fight or flight response, 23–24
finger stroking, 84–85, 115–116
finishing stroke, 58–59, 70
The Firelight Foundation (nonprofit
    organization), 237
fireplace, 185
five-minute massage, 175–176
flexibility, 107
floor, 50
flu, 189–190
folic acid, 209
fontanel, 87–88
foot massage
    Ankles Away technique, 68–69
    Chinese medicine, 69
    Let's Go sequence, 165, 166
    overview, 63–64
    This Little Piggy technique, 69–70
football hold, 183
forehead, 94–101
formula feeding
    constipation, 180
    digestion, 72
    feeding schedule, 141
    HIV-infected mother, 230
    past views, 8
foster child, 204–205, 206
Foundation for Healthy Living
    (massage resources), 248
Free to Be . . . You and Me
    (music CD), 149
friction, 12, 13
front carrier, 120
frustration, 39, 184
fussy baby
    cause, 192
    Chinese massage, 242
    compassion of parent, 30
    emotional development, 34–35
    first massage, 56
    overstimulation signs, 54
    overview, 192
    signs of stress, 24
    tips for soothing, 193
*The Fussy Baby Book: Parenting
    Your High-Need Child from
    Birth to Age Five* (Sears, William
    and Sears, Martha), 35

• G •

games, 150
gas, 72–76
gastroesophageal reflux disease
    (GERD), 182
gluteus maximi, 112–116
Goodnight Moon (Brown, Margaret
    Wise), 150
Gookin, Dan (*Parenting For
    Dummies*), 31
Gookin, Sandra Harding (*Parenting
    For Dummies*), 31
grounded baby, 141

• H •

Hale House (nonprofit
    organization), 222
hamstring, 108
hand containment, 135
hand massage
    Alternating Hands technique, 81
    cautions, 84
    finger stroking, 84–85
    five-minute massage, 175
    hand stroking, 84
    overview, 81, 83–84
hand washing, 235
*The Handbook of Chinese Massage
    Massage: Tui Na Techniques
    to Awaken Body and Mind*
    (Mercati, Maria), 243
Hanlon, Grace M. (*Successfully
    Parenting Your Baby with Special
    Needs: Early Intervention for
    Ages Birth to Three*), 237

hara, 48–49
hatching, 39
headache, 233
head-banging, 214–215
health problem. *See also specific
    problems*
  abdominal massage, 72
  benefits of massage, 16–17
  chest massage, 77
  Down syndrome complications,
    210, 211
  endorphins, 18
  injured baby, 55
hearing loss, 100
hearing screening test, 139
Heart Stroke, 77–78
High Contact Massage, 195
high need baby, 194–195
*HIV and AIDS in Mothers and
    Babies: A Guide to Counseling*
    (Sherr, Lorraine), 238
HIV-exposed baby
  benefits of massage, 12
  complementary therapies, 234
  massage techniques, 232–234
  medical tests, 230–231
  overview, 228
  resources, 237–238
  symptoms, 231–232
  transmission prevention, 228–230
  universal precautions, 234–235
holding baby, 15, 30, 35
holistic practice, 16–17
homeopathic remedy, 189
homeostasis, 13
homocysteine, 209
hospital
  bonding, 19–20, 34, 136
  newborn baby, 138–140
  premature baby, 133–136
  rooming in, 140
  routine tests, 139
humidifier, 196, 197

hungry baby, 54
Hyland's teething tablets, 189
hypertonia, 208
hypotonia, 208

• *I* •

I Love You stroke, 75–76
illness. *See* ailment
immune system
  benefits of massage, 29
  breastfeeding benefits, 142
  Chinese medicine, 29
  essential oils, 53
  HIV-infected baby, 231
incubator, 133, 134, 135
independence, 10
Indian culture, 11, 241–242
infant. *See also* newborn baby
  adoption, 202–203
  attention while massaging,
    145–146
  bathing tips, 171–172
  benefits of massage, 16
  diaper change, 174
  knowledge about, 22
  massage opportunities, 146–147
  naps, 163
  overview, 145
  readiness cues, 46
  rhymes, 147–148
infant development. *See also
    specific types*
  benefits of massage, 27–30
  delays, 206–216
  failure to thrive syndrome, 138
  overview, 31–32
  6 months to 1 year, 41–43, 146
  sleep, 162
  solid foods, 180
  spine, 116
  stages, 33
  3 to 6 months, 38–40

infant massage benefits
  ailments, 16–17
  bonding, 19–21
  depression, 12, 26–27
  developmental delays, 207–208
  drug-addicted baby, 221
  fathers, 22
  newborn development,
      16, 27–30
  parental skills, 21–22
  premature baby, 15
  research findings, 12
  stressed baby, 17, 22–26
  toddler, 16
Infant Massage (McClure,
    Vimala), 11
infant massage preparation
  first massage, 55–59
  location of massage, 49–50
  mood, 45–46, 51–53
  oil selection, 50–51
  safety, 50
  stress, 45–46
  timing, 49, 54–55
infant swing, 183
influenza, 190
injury, 55
insecurely attached baby, 201
insecurity, 22
Institute for Attachment & Child
    Development, 206
intention, 14–15, 46
interdependence, 10
international adoption, 203–204
International Association of Infant
    Massage, 11, 249
International Chiropractic Pediatric
    Association, 124
International Loving Touch
    Foundation, 249
intuition, 9, 55

• *J* •

Japanese massage, 243
jaw massage, 88–91
jewelry, 50
Johari, Harish (*Ayurvedic Massage:
    Traditional Indian Techniques for
    Balancing Body and Mind*), 242
joint motion, 12

• *K* •

kangaroo care, 135–136
karotype, 209
Kiehl's Baby Nurturing Cream for
    Face and Body, 197
kiss, 153
Kneading Dough technique,
    65–66, 110

• *L* •

La Leche League (breastfeeding
    resource), 202
lactic acid, 13
Large Bottom Stroke, 114–115
Lather, Patricia Ann (*Troubling the
    Angels: Women Living with
    HIV/AIDS*), 238
lavender, 53
laziness, 9
Leg Cross stretch, 244–245
leg massage
  Ankles Away technique, 68–69, 112
  backs of legs, 108–112
  five-minute massage, 175
  Kneading Dough technique,
      65–66, 110
  Let's Go sequence, 165–166
  Little Sleeper sequence, 164–165

overview, 63–64
premature baby, 137
raking, 70–71
safety, 110
Sleeper sequence, 164
Squeeze and Twist technique,
    66–67
Taffy Pull technique, 64–65, 110
Thumb Circles technique,
    67–68, 110
let-down reflex, 20
Let's Go sequence, 165–167
lighting, 34, 56, 137
Ling, Per Henrik (Father of
    Massage), 11
Little Forest (skin care product
    retailer), 248
Little Sleeper sequence, 164–165
Long Effleurage Stroke, 118–119
Long Stroke, 126–127
lotion, 197
low viral load, 230
lullaby music, 52
lymph fluid, 13

• *M* •

massage. *See specific types*
mattress, 36
McClure, Vimala (*Infant
    Massage*), 11
mediator, 184
medication, 36, 229, 232–233
mental retardation (MR), 213–216
Mercati, Maria (*The Handbook of
    Chinese Massage: Tui Na
    Techniques to Awaken Body
    and Mind*), 243
meridians, 69, 213

Mind/Body Institute (nonprofit
    organization), 238
mirror, 147
mixed cerebral palsy, 212
mood, 45–46, 51–53
mother
    alcoholism, 224
    benefits of massage, 134
    drug addiction, 220–221
    fetal alcohol syndrome
        support, 228
    frustration with colicky baby, 184
    high need baby tips, 195
    HIV-infected, 228–230
    kangaroo care, 136
    resources for support, 35
*The Mother's Survival Guide to
    Recovery: All About Alcohol,
    Drugs & Babies* (Tanner,
    Laurie), 237
motor development, 40, 41–42
mouthing, 147
MR (mental retardation), 213–216
muscle tone, 208–216
music
    head-banging remedy, 215
    massage preparation, 51–52, 56
    toddler massage, 149
myelin sheath, 28–29
myelinization, 28–29

• *N* •

Najavits, Lisa M. (*A Woman's
    Addiction Workbook: Your
    Guide to In-Depth Healing*), 237
nap, 161–168
National Dissemination Center for
    Children with Disabilities, 235

National Organization of Fetal
Alcohol Syndrome
(NOFAS), 228
National SIDS/Infant Death
Resource Center, 167
National Toxicology Program Center
for the Evaluation of Risks to
Human Reproduction, 236
*Natural Family Living: The Mother
Magazine Guide to Parenting*
(O'Mara, Peggy), 156
neck, 104–106, 126–127
neonatal intensive care unit (NICU),
133, 221
neurological development, 28–29
newborn baby. *See also* infant;
premature baby
  adoption, 201–202
  bathing tips, 169–170
  benefits of massage, 16, 27–30
  diaper change, 172–174
  hospital stay, 138–140
  increased massage techniques, 143
  massage schedule, 140–141
  naps, 162
NICU (neonatal intensive care unit),
133, 221
*The No-Cry Sleep Solution: Gentle
Ways to Help Your Baby
Sleep Through the Night*
(Pantley, Elizabeth), 162
NOFAS (National Organization of
Fetal Alcohol Syndrome), 228
noise, 33, 34
nonverbal communication, 21
nursery rhyme, 52, 147, 149
nursing. *See* breastfeeding
nurturing touch program, 133, 136
*Nutrition and HIV: A New Model for
Treatment* (Romeyn, Mary), 238
nutrition therapy, 234

• *O* •

oil
  application steps, 56
  premature baby, 137
  safety tips, 50
  scalp massage, 197–198
  selection, 50–51
  skin problems, 196
older baby. *See* infant
O'Mara, Peggy (*Natural Family
Living: The Mother Magazine
Guide to Parenting*), 156
Open Book Stroke, 78–79, 94–96
organized baby, 135
orphanage, 204
overstimulation
  back massage, 118
  clothing, 140
  drug-addicted baby, 222
  emotional development, 32–33
  overview, 54–55
  parent's response, 56
  premature baby, 136, 137–138
  Squeeze and Twist technique, 66
  stroke combinations, 71
  Thumb Circles technique, 67
  tips for avoiding, 160–161
oxycodone, 220
oxytocin, 20, 139

• *P* •

painkiller, 18
Pantley, Elizabeth (*The No-Cry
Sleep Solution: Gentle Ways
to Help Your Baby Sleep
Through the Night*), 162
parasympathetic nervous system,
23, 24
parent. *See* father; mother

Parenting For Dummies
(Gookin, Sandra Harding
and Gookin, Dan), 31
parenting skills
massage benefits, 21–22
perfection, 39
toddler, 152–154
PCR (polymerase chain reaction)
test, 230–231
peppermint oil, 191
peristalsis, 28
Perkins, Sharon (*Breastfeeding
For Dummies*), 72
person permanence, 41
Peter, Paul, & Mommy
(music CD), 149
petrissage stroke, 12, 65, 226
physical therapy, 212
placenta previa, 132
play, 38, 39–40
pollen, 184
polymerase chain reaction (PCR)
test, 230–231
positive authority, 155–156
posterior fontanel, 88
postpartum depression, 12, 26–27
posture
massage benefits, 116
massage preparation, 48–49
sitting, 245–246
power struggle, 153, 154, 163
preeclampsia, 132
pregnancy
history, 7
HIV-infected mother, 228–230
prenatal massage, 14
risks of premature labor, 132
premature baby. *See also* newborn
baby
back massage, 137
benefits of massage, 12, 15, 133–134

bonding, 133, 134
breastfeeding, 134, 142
eye contact, 137
hospital contact, 133–136
increased massage
techniques, 143
leg massage, 137
muscle tone, 208
overstimulation, 136, 137–138
overview, 131
special care needs, 133
stress, 132
tips for successful home massage,
136–138
prenatal massage, 14
preparation, infant massage
first massage, 55–59
location of massage, 49–50
mood, 45–46, 51–53
oil selection, 50–51
safety, 50
stress, 45–46
timing, 49, 54–55
pressure
amount, 47
Thumbs to Sides technique, 74
tickling, 64
Water Wheel technique, 73
preventative medicine, 17

• *R* •

Raking technique, 70–71, 125–126
rash, 196–197
reactive attachment disorder,
205–206
readiness cues, 46
reading, 149–150
reflection, 147
reflexology, 69
relationship building, 38

relaxation
  consistency of massage, 25
  nonverbal communication, 21
  response, 26, 47–48
respect, 152
restaurant, 176
ritual, 174–175
rivalry, sibling, 217
rocking baby, 13, 30
Romeyn, Mary (*Nutrition and HIV: A New Model for Treatment*), 238
rooming in, 140
routine
  bathing, 168–172
  diaper change, 172–174
  emotional development, 33–34, 36–37
  fetal alcohol syndrome, 226
  five-minute massage, 175–176
  increased massage, 143
  massage location, 176
  massage preparation tips, 49
  massage time selection, 159–160
  nap, 161–168
  newborn's routine, 140–141
  rituals, 174–175
rubber bulb syringe, 191
rules, 154–155
runner's high, 18
Ryan, Constance (*Children with HIV/AIDS*), 238

• S •

Sacral Stroke, 124–125
sacrum, 116, 124–125
safety
  allergic reaction, 51
  bathing, 169, 170
  co-sleeping, 36
  eyes, 93–94
  facial massage, 87–88

injured limbs, 55
leg massage, 110
massage preparation, 50
neck massage, 105
oil, 50
sibling massage, 151
spine, 116
scalp massage, 197–198
schedule
  bathing, 168–172
  diaper change, 172–174
  emotional development, 33–34, 36–37
  fetal alcohol syndrome, 226
  five-minute massage, 175–176
  increased massage, 143
  massage location, 176
  massage preparation tips, 49
  massage time selection, 159–160
  nap, 161–168
  newborn's routine, 140–141
  rituals, 174–175
scooping, 105–106
Sears, Martha and William
  The Discipline Book: How to Have a Better-Behaved Child from Birth to Age Ten, 156
  The Fussy Baby Book: Parenting Your High-Need Child from Birth to Age Five, 35
  Web site, 248
seborrhea, 197
securely attached baby, 200–201
seizure, 212
self-soothing skills, 30, 206
Sendak, Maurice (*Where the Wild Things Are*), 150
sensory awareness, 29
separation anxiety, 41, 42–43
separation individuation, 39, 40
sexual abuse, 153
shaken baby, 184

shaking, 25
shampoo, 169, 196
Sherr, Lorraine (*HIV and AIDS in Mothers and Babies: A Guide to Counseling*), 238
Shiatsu massage, 243
shoulder massage
 headache relief, 233
 Let's Go technique, 166, 167
 Long Stroke, 126–127
 overview, 76
siblings, 151, 216–217
side effects, 232–233
SIDS (sudden infant death syndrome), 36, 167
sign language, 215
Singable Songs for the Very Young (music CD), 149
singing
 bonding with premature baby, 134
 massage preparation, 52
 toddler massage, 147–148, 149
sinus congestion, 189–191, 211
sitting posture, 48, 245–246
skin problems, 196–198, 211
sleep
 adopted infant, 203, 204
 co-sleeping tips, 36, 167
 cycles, 162
 gentle waking techniques, 168
 high need baby, 194
 infant development, 162
 naps, 161–168
 SIDS prevention, 167
 signs of sleepiness, 163
 Taffy Pull technique, 64
 toddler, 150
Sleeper sequence, 164
sling, 15, 120, 183
slouching, 116
Small Circles technique
 back massage, 122–123
 facial massage, 89–90, 104–105

smile, 38, 168
Smile Stroke, 91–92
Smithies, Chris (*Troubling the Angels: Women Living with HIV/AIDS*), 238
smoking, 185
soap, 169, 170, 196
social development, 38–39
soft spot, 87–88
soft tissue, 13
solar plexus, 48–49
solid food, 180
sound machine, 52
spastic cerebral palsy, 211
speech therapy, 212
spine, 116–117, 124
spit up, 54, 72, 180
spoiled children, 10–11
spondylolisthesis, 120
Squeeze and Twist technique, 66–67
standing, 107
startle response, 24
stomach. *See* abdominal massage
stress
 asthma, 185
 benefits of massage, 17, 22–26
 breathing, 25, 184–185
 cause, 23–24
 colicky baby, 184
 digestive problems, 28
 effects, 24
 endorphins, 18
 exercise for parents, 25–26
 infant massage preparation, 45–46
 management tips, 30
 overview, 22–23
 premature baby, 132
 symptoms, 24–25
stretching, 243–245
stroke, 12–13, 71. *See also specific types*

subluxation, 124
Successfully Parenting Your Baby with Special Needs: Early Intervention for Ages Birth to Three (Hanlon, Grace M.), 237
sudden infant death syndrome (SIDS), 36, 167
Sun and Moon technique, 74–75
supermarket, 176
support group, 35, 184, 228
supported sitting, 245
swaddling, 34–35, 223
Swedish massage, 11–17
swing, infant, 183
Swooping technique, 121–122
sympathetic nervous system, 23

• T •

Taffy Pull technique, 64–65, 110
Tafuri, Nancy (*Will You Be My Friend? A Bunny and Bird Story*), 150
Tanner, Laurie (*The Mother's Survival Guide to Recovery: All About Alcohol, Drugs & Babies*), 237
tantrum, 156–157
tapotement stroke, 12, 13
Taylor-Brown, Susan (*Children with HIV/AIDS*), 238
tea tree oil, 53
teething
  breastfeeding, 188
  onset, 187
  overview, 40, 186
  signs, 187
  techniques for relief, 89–90, 188–189
temper tantrum, 156–157
Temple Stroke, 99, 101
This Little Piggy technique, 69–70
thoracic spine, 116
Thumb Circles technique, 67–68, 83, 110
Thumbs to Sides technique, 73–74

thumb-sucking, 30
tickling, 64
time
  knowledge of baby, 22
  massage preparation, 49
  quality versus quantity, 7–8
toddler
  benefits of massage, 16
  development, 148–149
  discipline, 152–157
  massage tips, 148–150
  overview, 148
  sleep, 150
toe massage, 69–70
tolerance, 47
touch
  benefits, 12
  bonding tips, 20
  emotional development, 35
  massage preparation, 46–47
  premature baby, 133–138
  sexual abuse, 153
touch relaxation technique, 71
Touch Research Institute (TRI), 12
towel, 197
toxic material, 13, 65
transcending colon, 72
transferential object, 202
trapezius muscle, 79
TRI (Touch Research Institute), 12
trigger point, 13
Troubling the Angels: Women Living with HIV/AIDS (Lather, Patricia Ann, and Smithies, Chris, 238
trust
  massage benefits, 20–21
  sexual abuse education, 153
  stress resilience, 30
  toddler discipline, 155
Tui Na massage (Chinese massage), 242–243
TV time, 152
twitching, 25

• *U* •

umbilical cord, 169
uncorking the bottle technique, 75
universal precautions, 234–235
The Upledger Institute (CranioSacral
    Therapy resource), 213
uterus, 142

• *V* •

vacation, 152
vaccination, 139
Vannais, Carol (*Breastfeeding
    For Dummies*), 72
vibration, 12
videos, 249–250
virus, 190
vitamin K shot, 139
vitamin therapy, 234
vomit, 54, 72

• *W* •

walking, 107
Water Wheel technique, 72–73
wearing baby, 15
Web sites
  acupuncture resources, 213
  basic resources, 247–248
  Bill and Martha Sears, 248
  breast milk storage, 134
  breastfeeding tips, 202
  children's music, 52, 147–148
  chiropractic care, 124
  CranioSacral Therapy, 213
  essential oils, 53

fetal alcohol syndrome, 228
Hale House, 222
HIV-exposed baby, 234, 238
massage associations, 248–249
parental support, 35, 228
reactive attachment disorder, 206
SIDS prevention, 167
sign language, 215
skin products, 197, 248
teething relief, 189
videos, 249
yoga, 234
Wei Chi (immune system), 29
weight gain, 28, 134, 225
Western culture, 11
*When Your Child Has a Disability:
    The Complete Sourcebook
    of Daily and Medical Care*
    (Batshaw, Mark L.), 236
Where the Wild Things Are
    (Sendak, Maurice), 150
white noise, 52
White-Gray, Myra (*Children
    with HIV/AIDS*), 238
*Will You Be My Friend? A Bunny and
    Bird Story* (Tafuri, Nancy), 150
withdrawal, drug, 220–221
*A Woman's Addiction Workbook:
    Your Guide to In-Depth Healing*
    (Najavits, Lisa M.), 237
wrist, 82, 83

• *Y* •

yoga, 234, 246, 250
Young Living Essential Oil
    (retailer), 53

Notes

BUSINESS, CAREERS & PERSONAL FINANCE

0-7645-5307-0   0-7645-5331-3 *†

Also available:

- Accounting For Dummies †
  0-7645-5314-3
- Business Plans Kit For Dummies †
  0-7645-5365-8
- Cover Letters For Dummies
  0-7645-5224-4
- Frugal Living For Dummies
  0-7645-5403-4
- Leadership For Dummies
  0-7645-5176-0
- Managing For Dummies
  0-7645-1771-6

- Marketing For Dummies
  0-7645-5600-2
- Personal Finance For Dummies *
  0-7645-2590-5
- Project Management
  For Dummies
  0-7645-5283-X
- Resumes For Dummies †
  0-7645-5471-9
- Selling For Dummies
  0-7645-5363-1
- Small Business Kit For Dummies *†
  0-7645-5093-4

HOME & BUSINESS COMPUTER BASICS

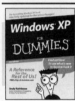

0-7645-4074-2   0-7645-3758-X

Also available:

- ACT! 6 For Dummies
  0-7645-2645-6
- iLife '04 All-in-One Desk Reference
  For Dummies
  0-7645-7347-0
- iPAQ For Dummies
  0-7645-6769-1
- Mac OS X Panther Timesaving
  Techniques For Dummies
  0-7645-5812-9
- Macs For Dummies
  0-7645-5656-8
- Microsoft Money 2004 For Dummies
  0-7645-4195-1

- Office 2003 All-in-One Desk
  Reference For Dummies
  0-7645-3883-7
- Outlook 2003 For Dummies
  0-7645-3759-8
- PCs For Dummies
  0-7645-4074-2
- TiVo For Dummies
  0-7645-6923-6
- Upgrading and Fixing PCs
  For Dummies
  0-7645-1665-5
- Windows XP Timesaving
  Techniques For Dummies
  0-7645-3748-2

FOOD, HOME, GARDEN, HOBBIES, MUSIC & PETS

0-7645-5295-3   0-7645-5232-5

Also available:

- Bass Guitar For Dummies
  0-7645-2487-9
- Diabetes Cookbook For Dummies
  0-7645-5230-9
- Gardening For Dummies *
  0-7645-5130-2
- Guitar For Dummies
  0-7645-5106-X
- Holiday Decorating For Dummies
  0-7645-2570-0
- Home Improvement All-in-One
  For Dummies
  0-7645-5680-0

- Knitting For Dummies
  0-7645-5395-X
- Piano For Dummies
  0-7645-5105-1
- Puppies For Dummies
  0-7645-5255-4
- Scrapbooking For Dummies
  0-7645-7208-3
- Senior Dogs For Dummies
  0-7645-5818-8
- Singing For Dummies
  0-7645-2475-5
- 30-Minute Meals For Dummies
  0-7645-2589-1

INTERNET & DIGITAL MEDIA

0-7645-1664-7   0-7645-6924-4

Also available:

- 2005 Online Shopping Directory
  For Dummies
  0-7645-7495-7
- CD & DVD Recording For Dummies
  0-7645-5956-7
- eBay For Dummies
  0-7645-5654-1
- Fighting Spam For Dummies
  0-7645-5965-6
- Genealogy Online For Dummies
  0-7645-5964-8
- Google For Dummies
  0-7645-4420-9

- Home Recording For Musicians
  For Dummies
  0-7645-1634-5
- The Internet For Dummies
  0-7645-4173-0
- iPod & iTunes For Dummies
  0-7645-7772-7
- Preventing Identity Theft
  For Dummies
  0-7645-7336-5
- Pro Tools All-in-One Desk
  Reference For Dummies
  0-7645-5714-9
- Roxio Easy Media Creator
  For Dummies
  0-7645-7131-1

* Separate Canadian edition also available
† Separate U.K. edition also available

Available wherever books are sold. For more information or to order direct: U.S. customers
visit www.dummies.com or call 1-877-762-2974.
U.K. customers visit www.wileyeurope.com or call 0800 243407. Canadian customers visit
www.wiley.ca or call 1-800-567-4797.

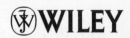

SPORTS, FITNESS, PARENTING, RELIGION & SPIRITUALITY

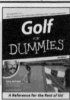
0-7645-5146-9

0-7645-5418-2

Also available:
- Adoption For Dummies
  0-7645-5488-3
- Basketball For Dummies
  0-7645-5248-1
- The Bible For Dummies
  0-7645-5296-1
- Buddhism For Dummies
  0-7645-5359-3
- Catholicism For Dummies
  0-7645-5391-7
- Hockey For Dummies
  0-7645-5228-7

- Judaism For Dummies
  0-7645-5299-6
- Martial Arts For Dummies
  0-7645-5358-5
- Pilates For Dummies
  0-7645-5397-6
- Religion For Dummies
  0-7645-5264-3
- Teaching Kids to Read
  For Dummies
  0-7645-4043-2
- Weight Training For Dummies
  0-7645-5168-X
- Yoga For Dummies
  0-7645-5117-5

TRAVEL

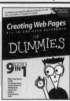
0-7645-5438-7

0-7645-5453-0

Also available:
- Alaska For Dummies
  0-7645-1761-9
- Arizona For Dummies
  0-7645-6938-4
- Cancún and the Yucatán
  For Dummies
  0-7645-2437-2
- Cruise Vacations For Dummies
  0-7645-6941-4
- Europe For Dummies
  0-7645-5456-5
- Ireland For Dummies
  0-7645-5455-7

- Las Vegas For Dummies
  0-7645-5448-4
- London For Dummies
  0-7645-4277-X
- New York City For Dummies
  0-7645-6945-7
- Paris For Dummies
  0-7645-5494-8
- RV Vacations For Dummies
  0-7645-5443-3
- Walt Disney World & Orlando
  For Dummies
  0-7645-6943-0

GRAPHICS, DESIGN & WEB DEVELOPMENT

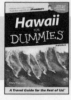
0-7645-4345-8

0-7645-5589-8

Also available:
- Adobe Acrobat 6 PDF
  For Dummies
  0-7645-3760-1
- Building a Web Site For Dummies
  0-7645-7144-3
- Dreamweaver MX 2004
  For Dummies
  0-7645-4342-3
- FrontPage 2003 For Dummies
  0-7645-3882-9
- HTML 4 For Dummies
  0-7645-1995-6
- Illustrator CS For Dummies
  0-7645-4084-X

- Macromedia Flash MX 2004
  For Dummies
  0-7645-4358-X
- Photoshop 7 All-in-One Desk
  Reference For Dummies
  0-7645-1667-1
- Photoshop CS Timesaving
  Techniques For Dummies
  0-7645-6782-9
- PHP 5 For Dummies
  0-7645-4166-8
- PowerPoint 2003 For Dummies
  0-7645-3908-6
- QuarkXPress 6 For Dummies
  0-7645-2593-X

NETWORKING, SECURITY, PROGRAMMING & DATABASES

0-7645-6852-3

0-7645-5784-X

Also available:
- A+ Certification For Dummies
  0-7645-4187-0
- Access 2003 All-in-One Desk
  Reference For Dummies
  0-7645-3988-4
- Beginning Programming
  For Dummies
  0-7645-4997-9
- C For Dummies
  0-7645-7068-4
- Firewalls For Dummies
  0-7645-4048-3
- Home Networking For Dummies
  0-7645-42796

- Network Security For Dummies
  0-7645-1679-5
- Networking For Dummies
  0-7645-1677-9
- TCP/IP For Dummies
  0-7645-1760-0
- VBA For Dummies
  0-7645-3989-2
- Wireless All In-One Desk Reference
  For Dummies
  0-7645-7496-5
- Wireless Home Networking
  For Dummies
  0-7645-3910-8

HEALTH & SELF-HELP

0-7645-6820-5 *†   0-7645-2566-2

Also available:

- Alzheimer's For Dummies
  0-7645-3899-3
- Asthma For Dummies
  0-7645-4233-8
- Controlling Cholesterol For Dummies
  0-7645-5440-9
- Depression For Dummies
  0-7645-3900-0
- Dieting For Dummies
  0-7645-4149-8
- Fertility For Dummies
  0-7645-2549-2

- Fibromyalgia For Dummies
  0-7645-5441-7
- Improving Your Memory For Dummies
  0-7645-5435-2
- Pregnancy For Dummies †
  0-7645-4483-7
- Quitting Smoking For Dummies
  0-7645-2629-4
- Relationships For Dummies
  0-7645-5384-4
- Thyroid For Dummies
  0-7645-5385-2

EDUCATION, HISTORY, REFERENCE & TEST PREPARATION

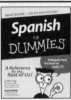

0-7645-5194-9   0-7645-4186-2

Also available:

- Algebra For Dummies
  0-7645-5325-9
- British History For Dummies
  0-7645-7021-8
- Calculus For Dummies
  0-7645-2498-4
- English Grammar For Dummies
  0-7645-5322-4
- Forensics For Dummies
  0-7645-5580-4
- The GMAT For Dummies
  0-7645-5251-1
- Inglés Para Dummies
  0-7645-5427-1

- Italian For Dummies
  0-7645-5196-5
- Latin For Dummies
  0-7645-5431-X
- Lewis & Clark For Dummies
  0-7645-2545-X
- Research Papers For Dummies
  0-7645-5426-3
- The SAT I For Dummies
  0-7645-7193-1
- Science Fair Projects For Dummies
  0-7645-5460-3
- U.S. History For Dummies
  0-7645-5249-X

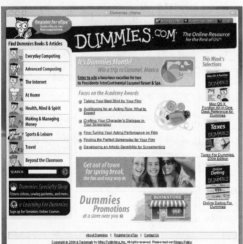

Get smart @ dummies.com®

- **Find a full list of Dummies titles**
- **Look into loads of FREE on-site articles**
- **Sign up for FREE eTips e-mailed to you weekly**
- **See what other products carry the Dummies name**
- **Shop directly from the Dummies bookstore**
- **Enter to win new prizes every month!**

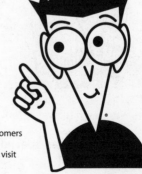

* Separate Canadian edition also available
† Separate U.K. edition also available

Available wherever books are sold. For more information or to order direct: U.S. customers visit www.dummies.com or call 1-877-762-2974.
U.K. customers visit www.wileyeurope.com or call 0800 243407. Canadian customers visit www.wiley.ca or call 1-800-567-4797.

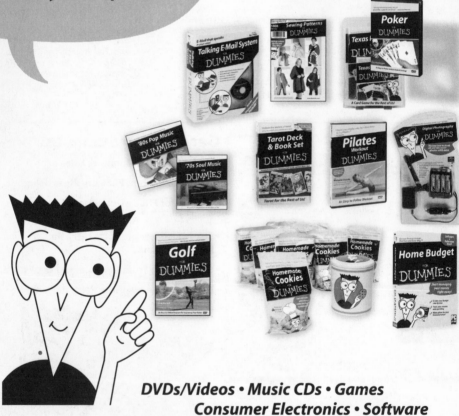
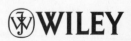